# The Ultimate Workout Log

# The Ultimate Workout Log

## An Exercise Diary for Everyone

### FOURTH EDITION

## SUZANNE SCHLOSBERG

HOUGHTON MIFFLIN HARCOURT

*Boston New York*

**To all the exercisers who have kept this log going**

**for nearly two decades**

www.hmhco.com

ISBN 978-0-547-59212-1

Printed in the United States of America

Book design by Lisa Diercks
Typeset in The Serif

13 2021
4500830170

# Contents

# WHAT'S NEW
# IN THE FOURTH EDITION?

I hope you enjoy this edition's improved layout!

The new format allows for longer comments on cardio and strength workouts, and more space to record changes in weight and reps from one set to the next. This edition lasts 26 weeks, two longer than previous editions, so you can track a full year of workouts in two logs. As always, you'll find fresh tips, inspirational quotes, and fitness factoids. Who runs faster: a world-class sprinter or a zebra? You'll find out in Week 7.

# Introduction to the Fourth Edition

While cleaning out a closet a while back, I unearthed a box of my old workout logs, more than two dozen. What fun!

The notations are sparse—"Skyliners, 39:06!" or "rode Latigo w/ Amy, 40 mi."—but they brought back so many people and places. Like the Nordic skier I dated who referred to himself and his skis as "we." (Log note: "Skied 10 mi. w/Weird Dave.") And the time I lied to my boyfriend, feigning a love for backpacking, then suffered through a 200-mile trek that I'd neglected to train for ("I'm an IDIOT"). Oh, and my first post-pregnancy trip to the gym ("OMG, abs?????"). I've always been too lazy to keep a personal journal, so it was a kick to discover that I'd done so without even trying.

A workout log is invaluable in more ways than you may imagine. These pages will prod you to set worthy goals and plan strategies to reach them, encourage you to stick to your program, and bring you a feeling of accomplishment. It doesn't matter whether you're a novice exerciser or an Olympian, whether you're aiming to drop 30 pounds or bench-press 300. Your log will help you get results. "The mere fact of writing something down makes you more committed to it," says the sports psychologist Robert Weinberg, Ph.D., a professor at Miami University in Ohio. "You try harder."

Of course, sometimes we try too hard, running ourselves ragged, and in those instances, your log will come in handy, too. Tracking your workouts—your times and distances, your intensity, your energy level, your sleep quality—is the best way to dissect and reflect on your training. "If you're tired or injured or not making progress, you can usually find the answer in your log," says Jerzy Gregorek, a four-time world weightlifting champion and head coach of the UCLA weightlifting team.

When you track your workouts for months and years, patterns emerge. Your log will reveal the strategies that work well for your body and your psyche, and those that leave you feeling wiped out or uninspired. "If you're not performing well, you feel like you need to work harder, harder, harder," the pro mountain biker Rebecca Rusch, a.k.a. the "Queen of Pain," told me. "But then you dig yourself into a bigger hole. A while back, my workouts and my sleep were suffering. My log made me realize I needed to back off."

It's so easy to forget what you did two days ago, let alone two weeks ago. Without records, you might perceive that you're working out five days a week when, in reality, you're averaging only two or three visits to the gym. A log keeps you honest and holds you accountable when you veer off course or toward the couch. "I'm just as guilty of sloth as the next person," says Rebecca, a three-time winner of the 24-hour solo world championship. (Sloth? Really?) She says she relies on her log notes and goals, along with her training partners, to get her psyched for her next workout.

A training diary helps you believe in yourself, reminding you of all the mileage you've banked, the effort you've expended, the progress you've made. Stair-climbing superwoman Melissa Moon, who has won the Empire State Building Run-Up (86 flights of stairs in 13 minutes, 13 seconds!) and Germany's Swissôtel Vertical Marathon (76 stories), has maintained training logs for 17 years. "I like to flip through my logs when I have an important race coming up," the New Zealander says. "I'll look at how I was feeling mentally leading up to the event before and my times for certain workouts. This can be a great confidence builder."

In this log, you'll track your workouts as well as your goals for each week and for the next six months. You'll also find a chart to list personal records (PRs)—not just big records, like a new personal best in a 10k run, but small ones, too, like the first time you held crow pose in yoga class. No record is too minor to celebrate! The Olympic weightlifter Natalie Burgener says she tracks "every imaginable PR"—from her best double power snatch to her best triple in the clean and jerk. "This way, I always have something to reach for, even when a competition is far off."

## LOGGING FOR WEIGHT LOSS

What if your goal is losing weight rather than lifting weight? The more often you record your workouts, the more pounds you're likely to drop, research shows.

Consider: In a six-month study, Rob Carels, Ph.D., a psychology professor at Ohio's Bowling Green State University, found that conscientious loggers lost nearly twice as much weight, 23 pounds compared to 12 pounds, as those who rarely filled in their logs. The regular notetakers exercised 174 minutes a week, compared to 89 minutes for the slacker trackers. In another study, Carels discovered that the successful losers—those who shed at least 5 percent of their body weight over three months—kept food and exercise diaries on 81 days, virtually every day of the study. Those who failed to meet the 5-percent goal tracked their habits on only 35 days.

"It's a pretty consistent phenomenon: If you're recording diligently, exercise becomes more habitual," Carels says. Maintaining your log can be the difference between success and stagnation.

Even the gymnast Shannon Miller, a seven-time Olympic medalist, used a log to shed weight she'd gained after retiring from competition. "It's amazing how quickly you can succeed if you have a black-

and-white reminder of the good and bad habits you have formed," she says.

And how's this for amazing: Amy Barnes, a mom of two who lives in Woodbridge, Virginia, lost 350 pounds in four and a half years. She credits her success, in large part, to the daily notes she made in her 4-by-6-inch journals. "At first my notes were like, 'I did my Tae Bo video for eight minutes and thought I was going to pass out' or 'Glad this week is over.' But as the weight came off, my notes became more and more positive, like 'Wow! Can't believe I did it!'"

These days Amy is a lean, powerful fitness trainer. She keeps her old logs, hundreds of them, in storage boxes at home and pulls them out when she needs a boost. "Sometimes it's hard to remember what it felt like to walk a block at 500 pounds. My logs put things into perspective, reminding me how hard it all was and that it was worth every single step."

My hope is that you find as much inspiration from your logs as Amy has from hers.

As always, I welcome your feedback.

**Suzanne Schlosberg**
suzanne@suzanneschlosberg.com

# Setting Goals

The Olympic weightlifter Natalie Burgener incorporates her goals into her passwords—on her computer, at the ATM, and so on—so that she thinks about those dream numbers even when she's not hoisting barbells over her head. The Nordic skier Kikkan Randall, a three-time Olympian, writes her biggest aspiration of the year on the air freshener in her car. "That way I can see it every day," Kikkan says. "I also put little visual cues, like the Olympic Rings, all around my house and my notebooks."

You achieve more when you set targets; athletes know it and research proves it. You're more motivated and committed when you step onto the track or the elliptical trainer with a sense of purpose than when you slog aimlessly through your routine. Rebecca Rusch, a champion mountain biker, says she used to "just go out and train," but the scattershot approach got her to only about 80 percent of her capabilities. Once she started training in pursuit of specific goals and logging her workouts, she got better and better. "At 42, I am fitter and faster than I have ever been," she reports.

This log devotes a lot of space to recording your goals and assessing whether you've reached them. Goal-setting can be a trial-and-error process, so consider the following tips as you note your aspirations.

## MAKE YOUR GOALS SPECIFIC AND MEASURABLE
"Without numbers to reach for, you have chaos," says the world-

champion weightlifter Jerzy Gregorek. "I'm constantly aware of the world record and how far I am from that. If somebody broke my record somewhere, that drives me and excites me. Setting goals makes you reach in your brain for a little bit more."

This applies even if you're not aiming for world-record lifts. For example, in a classic three-month study conducted at Miami University in Ohio, researchers told a group of exercisers that their goal was to increase by 20 percent the number of abdominal crunches they could do. They told a second group simply, "Do your best." Not surprisingly, the group with the concrete objective performed 10 percent better than their rudderless peers. Along the same lines, in a review of 26 studies published in the *Journal of the American Medical Association,* researchers found that pedometer users increased their daily step count by 27 percent, about 2,200 steps per day, over about four months. The pedometer wearers who had the most success were those who set a specific goal, such as taking 10,000 steps per day.

Even if your ultimate goals aren't easy to quantify—maybe you're striving to be slimmer or healthier or feel more energetic—choose specific objectives to guide your training. You could aim to complete a 100-mile bike ride or run 30 minutes on the treadmill at a 9-minute-per-mile pace or take a core class twice a week for a month.

### MAKE YOUR GOALS CHALLENGING YET REALISTIC
Some people get fired up by goals that seem farfetched; they rise to the occasion and overachieve, says the sports psychologist Robert Weinberg. "But others will say, 'To hell with it. I'm outta here!' There's a lot of individual difference." In one study, researchers gave subjects a seemingly impossible goal: improve their sit-up performance by 60 repetitions over three months. Thirty percent of the subjects actually met the goal. Others, however, became demoralized and lost motivation to train.

Figure out what type of goals suit your personality. For most people, moderately difficult goals—those that are challenging but not pie-in-the-sky—work well. "I'm realistic—I'm not going to lie to myself," says the champion mountain biker Rebecca Rusch. "But if you choose safe goals that you know you can accomplish already, achieving them is not that rewarding. It's good to push outside the envelope and surprise yourself."

Amy Barnes, a fitness trainer who once weighed 500 pounds, took a more modest approach to goal setting. "I'd walk around the block and every week, I'd add one block," she recalls. "The first time it took me a whole hour to get around the block. The next week I'd try to do it in less than 60 minutes." She lost her first 100 pounds doing videos at home; each week, her goal increased by one minute.

## SET LONG-TERM, SHORT-TERM, AND "MICRO-TERM" GOALS

"I have two objectives that I operate from: the short-term goals and the 'things I need to do before I die' list," says the legendary ultramarathoner Tim Twietmeyer, a five-time winner of the grueling 100-mile Western States Endurance Run. "The short-term goals drive what I do day to day, and the other list drives my planning for bigger, more outrageous efforts that I want to complete."

Even if you feel your life would be complete without snowshoeing for 26 hours over the Sierra Nevada Mountains—as Twietmeyer and some friends did, becoming the first to cross the Sierra on foot since the 1850s—his philosophy is a wise one.

Long-term goals, like running a marathon next year or completing a cycling tour of the Napa Valley wine country, will get your juices flowing, but you also need to establish stepping stones. Smaller, more immediate goals will keep you on track and make your dream goals achievable. Set goals to accomplish every six or eight weeks, as well as weekly goals and even daily goals.

"The most important lesson I learned over the years was to set an intention for every training session," says the cross-country skier Beckie

Scott, who won Olympic gold for Canada. "My coach used to say that you don't hand in your training log at the start line. In other words, if winning races were a matter of just putting in the hours, anybody could do it. The difference is in how you approach those hours, training with a specific purpose every time you go out there."

Your purpose needn't be hardcore, says Jayne Williams, author of *Shape Up with the Slow Fat Triathlete*. "When you're starting out, you need micro-term goals, like 'I'm going to ride my bike to the park because I'll feel better.' Get used to sweating a little before you work up to sweating a lot. Otherwise you're going to start fearing your next workout like a root canal without Novocain."

### FOCUS ON A FEW GOALS

Don't set too many targets. Sure, most of us strive to become stronger, more flexible, and more consistent about exercise, and to have more stamina. But anyone who tries to achieve all of these objectives at once will go bonkers. Assess your priorities and focus on reaching the goals that are most important to you right now.

### FOCUS ON "PROCESS" RATHER THAN "OUTCOME" GOALS

This is just sports-psychology jargon for saying that you should focus on things you can control rather than those you can't. For example, even if you are determined to lose weight, don't write in your log, "Goal: lose twelve pounds in eight weeks." That objective may be concrete and measurable, and it may even be realistic, but it's not necessarily within your control. Even if two overweight people follow the exact same eating plan and workout program, they're not going to lose precisely the same amount of weight. Some bodies hang on to calories more easily than others.

So choose objectives like "lift weights three days a week" or "compete in two 10ks." Even if some of your goals are connected to a specific outcome, like completing a two-day breast-cancer walkathon or finishing in the top ten in a bike race, have backup goals you can feel good about in case life gets in the way of achieving your dream goals.

## DEVELOP STRATEGIES TO ACHIEVE YOUR GOALS

Setting goals isn't worth much without a plan to get you to your destination. Completing an Olympic-distance triathlon might be well within your abilities, but if you don't know how to split your workout time among running, biking, and swimming or how best to vary your intensity level, you may not get the results you're seeking. Whether your goals are modest or lofty, consider hiring a trainer or coach to help you devise a plan, or find a plan online.

Even the simplest goals require strategizing. For example, if you're aiming to exercise four days a week, examine the obstacles that have hindered you in the past and make some changes. Maybe you need to join a gym with childcare, or join a club close to your office, or wake up a half hour earlier to exercise, or find a workout buddy in your neighborhood.

Training plans aren't all it takes to achieve your goals. Says the Olympic gold medalist Nordic skier Chandra Crawford: "Great goals can still fall by the wayside if you don't build in the necessary support, fun, and friendship to keep it going when you get tired, busy, or just plain don't feel like training."

## BE FLEXIBLE

"Goals are a starting place, they're not ending places," says sports psychologist Weinberg. "Stuff happens, things change, and sometimes you have to reevaluate." Whatever goals you set, don't be a slave to them. If your training isn't going according to plan—if you get injured or sidetracked by a major work project, or if you're just not performing as well as you'd expected—cut yourself some slack. Cross out the old ones and pencil in new ones.

# Filling In Your Log

This is *your* log; you can scribble all over it or leave plenty of blanks. Some people thrive on minutiae; others are more partial to broad strokes.

The amount of information you track probably will vary with your mood and training goals. When you're gunning for a personal best in a competition, you may want to keep detailed records, noting your morning heart rate, pre-exercise snack, energy level before and during your workout, and so on. When you're in a lull, you may simply want to write "Swam."

Even if you record minimal data, note *something* every day, including the days you don't exercise. This way, when you look back, you'll be able to distinguish between days you intentionally rested, days you were sick or injured, and days when you blew off a planned workout. If you find yourself recording too many zeroes, ask yourself why. Did you run out of time? Were you too tired? Use your log to figure out what your hurdles are and how much training your body can handle.

The following are tips for filling out each section of your log. Soon you'll develop your own system.

## FILLING IN YOUR GOALS FOR THE NEXT SIX MONTHS
The log's inside cover is the place to consider the big picture: your cur-

rent fitness level and lifestyle habits, and what you'd like to accomplish over the next 26 weeks. You'll find a sample on page 13.

I think six months is the perfect time frame for setting long-term goals: It's close enough to make your goals feel attainable, yet far enough in the future to allow for making major progress. At the end of 26 weeks, flip back to this page and see how your results match up with your goals. You'll be thrilled at how far you've come.

In the Overall Goals section, note the one really big thing you want to achieve, along with two lesser goals. Often, achieving one major fitness goal requires improving in several areas, such as eating more healthfully, dropping a few pounds, or gaining leg strength. In other cases, you may be focused purely on one component of fitness and then be delighted to discover that, along the way, you gained strength or lost weight.

Whatever your aspirations, fill in the Starting Point section for each category—Cardio, Strength, and so on—recording details about your current abilities, exercise frequency, body measurements, eating habits, even feelings about working out. Fill in the Goals spaces where appropriate. You may find it distracting or overwhelming to set goals in all categories at once. And in some categories, setting precise goals isn't practical. For example, body-fat percentage—the percentage of your body that is composed of fat, as opposed to bones, organs, connective tissue, and blood—improves when you lose fat. But since that number depends partly on the weight of your muscle, bones, and organs, you can't simply pick a target and expect to nail it precisely. The same goes for your resting heart rate, which is the number of times your heart beats per minute when you're not moving. This number is largely genetically determined, but if you train regularly for six months, chances are your resting heart rate will decrease.

## USING YOUR DAILY LOG

The following are ideas for filling out each section of the daily diary.

## GOALS FOR THE WEEK

You can set your weekly goals in terms of distance ("Jog 15 miles" or "walk 10,000 steps/day"), time ("5 hrs total cardio"), or number of sessions ("Pilates 2x/swim 3x").

Though it's important to pick concrete targets, keep in mind that not all worthy goals involve numbers. You might aim to become a more skilled descender on your mountain bike or to let loose in your Zumba class. If you plan to push hard some weeks, balance out your program with easy weeks, too. Many athletes schedule three successively more challenging weeks followed by a recovery week in which they cut their distance and intensity by 25 percent to 50 percent.

## MORNING INFO

You can use the Morning Info box to record any number of markers. For example:

⏩ Hours slept or sleep quality. Sleep deprivation can zap your energy, concentration, and good humor and throw off your appetite-regulating hormones, making it tough to lose weight.

⏩ Weight. Daily weighing is a proven weight-control tool, helping you nip a problem in the bud. If you wait a month to weigh yourself, you might discover that, oops, you've gained five pounds! Your weight will naturally vary from day to day, so focus on the big picture. (Track your weight loss using the chart on pages 230–31.)

⏩ How you felt, physically or emotionally, when you woke up. Over time you may notice a connection between your morning mood and the quality of your workouts.

⏩ Resting heart rate. A higher-than-normal resting heart rate can signal that you're overtraining in general or haven't recovered from

# Sample Goals for the Next Six Months

➡ **OVERALL GOALS**

1. Run ¹/2 marathon
2. Improve balance—do yoga 2x/week
3. Cut back on sugar

➡ **CARDIO GOALS**

Starting Point Running 3 days/week, 3–4 miles, about 9:30 pace

Goals Join ¹/2-marathon training program, find running buddies, do speed work

➡ **STRENGTH GOALS**

Starting Point Yoga 1x week, no weights

Goals Stick w/yoga for now, increase to 2x

➡ **BALANCE AND FLEXIBILITY GOALS**

Starting Point "Yoga for runners" 1x/week—lousy balance and hamstring flexibility

Goals Yoga 2x/week, try power yoga class, nail Bird of Paradise and Side Crow

➡ **NUTRITION GOALS**

Starting Point Too much sugar, nighttime snacking

Goals Only fruit after dinner, cut back on vanilla pumps in latte

➡ **BODY GOALS**

| CURRENT | Weight 154 | Body fat% 26 | Resting HR 55 |
| --- | --- | --- | --- |
| Chest 40 in. | Waist 34 | Hips 41.5  Thighs 25 | Arms 14 |

| GOAL WEIGHT | 148 |
| --- | --- |

| SIX MONTHS | Weight | Body fat% | Resting HR |
| --- | --- | --- | --- |
| Chest | Waist | Hips  Thighs | Arms |

the previous day's workout and need a rest day. Keeping a heart-rate monitor on your nightstand makes it easy to get an accurate read first thing in the morning.

## DAILY RATING

Although the Daily Rating box is at the top of the page, fill out this intensity rating after your workout. Rate your workouts on a scale from 1 to 5 based on how hard you pushed your body. A 1 rating would be a super-easy day; a 5 would be a killer workout. Shoot for a healthy mix of numbers. Log a 0 for days you don't exercise.

Each week, transfer your daily ratings to the chart on page 232, titled "Workout Ratings: The Big Picture." At a glance, you can see that it's been two weeks since you took a day off or did a workout rated lower than 3, and maybe that's why you're feeling so wiped out. Or maybe it's been five days since you exercised at all!

## CARDIO EXERCISE

Here you can record up to three different activities, including how many minutes or hours you exercised, the distance you covered, and your intensity. Use the Cardio Notes section below to note extras, such as how you felt before, during, and/or after your workout, your route, your workout partners, the instructor of your class or video, or the weather.

You might notice, for example, that you cycle up a certain hill much faster when you ride with Lisa than when you're with Dave. (This may be good or bad; if you're toast after those Lisa rides, you might call Dave more often.) Or you can give yourself an extra pat on the back for completing a certain jogging course in the rain.

Say you warmed up on the elliptical trainer for 10 minutes on level 4. Then you did a 25-minute treadmill workout: 20 minutes of intervals at 5.5 mph, alternating 1 minute at a 2.0 incline and 3 minutes without an incline, followed by a 5-minute cool-down. You might write:

| CARDIO EXERCISE | TIME/DISTANCE/INTENSITY |
| --- | --- |
| Elliptical | 10 min., L4 easy |
| Treadmill | 25 min. total: 20 min. of intervals |
| | 5.5 mph—alt. 1 min. 2.0 incline/ |
| **Cardio Notes** | 3 min. flat; 5-min. cool-down |
| Hills tough but finished strong | |

## STRENGTH TRAINING

Here you can record up to 3 sets of 10 strength-training exercises. For each set, note how much weight you lifted and the number of repetitions you performed. If you're a beginner, it's especially helpful to write down the names of the exercises. Noting "lat pulldown" will reinforce the notion that the exercise is primarily a back (*latissimus dorsi*) exercise rather than an arm strengthener. If you don't know the name of a particular exercise, ask a trainer at your gym or search online. The American Council on Exercise, www.acefitness.org, has an extensive library of strength-training exercises.

Use the Strength Notes section below to comment on how you felt on a lift ("Strong bench press today!") or how you felt in general ("Struggled, quit early").

Let's say you did three sets of biceps curls: First 10 reps of 12 pounds, then 8 reps of 15 pounds, then 7 reps of 15 pounds. Then you did three sets of crunches on a physioball.

| STRENGTH TRAINING | Weight | Reps | Weight | Reps | Weight | Reps |
| --- | --- | --- | --- | --- | --- | --- |
| Biceps curls | 12 | 10 | 15 | 8 | 15 | 7 |
| Ball crunches | | 12 | | 12 | | 12 |
| | | | | | | |
| | | | | | | |
| **Strength Notes** | | | | | | |
| Felt weak from the get-go so didn't push | | | | | | |

## BALANCE AND FLEXIBILITY

Whether you're 20 or 80, a regimen of stretching and balance exercises will make you a better athlete, improve your posture, help you move more gracefully, and prevent falls and back pain. Yet these are the components of fitness we're most likely to blow off. This box is a reminder to stretch and work on your balance, whether you do yoga, Pilates, the Wii Balance Board, or simple stretches and balance moves at the park.

For example:

Power vinyasa yoga w/Phyllis—sweatfest!

Felt flexible today

## NUTRITION NOTES

You can use this box to monitor your eating habits in countless ways. Just keep in mind that this log is not intended as a food diary. (To track your eating habits in detail, check out *The Ultimate Diet Log*.)

Rather than record every cookie you eat, use the Nutrition Notes space to focus on one or two nutrition goals at a time. For instance, record how many vegetables you ate in a day, or note when you made a particularly wise food choice, like "ate turkey on whole wheat instead of Big Mac." You could record your breakfast choices for a week straight with the goal of boosting your fiber intake and cutting back on sugary cereals or muffins. For a nutrient breakdown of just about any food, go to the U.S. Department of Agriculture's National Nutrient Database for Standard Reference, www.nal.usda.gov/fnic/foodcomp/search/ or websites such as www.calorieking.com, www.caloriecount.about.com, or www.thecaloriecounter.com.

To see how your eating habits affect your exercise performance, try recording what you eat before exercising, and look for trends. Maybe you tend to finish stronger on a two-hour bike ride when you eat a bagel with peanut butter than when you eat a plain bagel. Or maybe you have more stamina for tennis when you eat 30 minutes before a match than when you eat two hours before.

**WEEKLY WRAP-UP**

Here's your opportunity to reflect on the week that just ended. Recording all that you accomplished one week will get you psyched as you start the next.

➡ Weekly Rating: This needn't be a precise average of your daily ratings, but use this 1-to-5 scale to record how hard you pushed your body during the week. Transfer your weekly ratings to the chart on page 232 titled "Workout Ratings: The Big Picture."

➡ Highlight of the Week: Use this line to note one specific accomplishment. It can be anything from "survived killer Spinning class" to "took a day off when I felt a cold coming on—smart!" If any of these highlights is particularly noteworthy, record it in the "Personal Records" chart on page 233.

➡ Goals: This section prompts you to look back at the goals you set the previous Monday. If you frequently exceed your goals, perhaps you need more of a challenge. If you consistently fall short, you may have unrealistic expectations; make a note about why you think you didn't meet your goals.

➡ Cardio Notes: Assess your week as a whole, and record whether you felt strong or below par. You can use the boxes to record how many days of the week you did cardio exercise, the total number of hours you spent working out, and, depending on your activity, your total mileage or swim yardage. Don't feel compelled to use all three boxes; some may not be relevant to you.

➡ Strength Notes: Jot down anything significant that happened on the strength-training front. In the Total Workouts space, note how many times you lifted weights or used other strength-training equipment, whether in a gym weight room, a studio strength class, or at home while following a video on your iPad. If you do a split routine (working different muscles on different days), you may want to use the space below to record how many days you worked each muscle group or body area. For instance, if you did two upper-body workouts but worked your legs and core only once, you might note: "upper: 2, lower: 1, core: 1."

➡ Balance and Flexibility Notes: Note how many times you stretched or worked on your balance (or took a class that included exercises for both), along with any feelings about the sessions or notes about your progress.

➡ Nutrition Notes: Record any patterns in your eating habits over the week. Maybe you chose nutritious snacks all week. Maybe you ate breakfast consistently, or perhaps you succumbed three times to that maple scone.

# Workout Diary

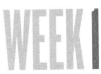WEEK 1

Dates _____

Goals _____
_____

# MONDAY

MORNING INFO [ ]    DAILY RATING [ ]

**CARDIO EXERCISE** _____    **TIME/DISTANCE/INTENSITY** _____

_____    _____

_____    _____

_____    _____

**Cardio Notes** _____

| STRENGTH TRAINING | Weight | Reps | Weight | Reps | Weight | Reps |
|---|---|---|---|---|---|---|
| _____ | | | | | | |
| _____ | | | | | | |
| _____ | | | | | | |
| _____ | | | | | | |
| _____ | | | | | | |
| _____ | | | | | | |
| _____ | | | | | | |
| _____ | | | | | | |
| _____ | | | | | | |
| _____ | | | | | | |

**Strength Notes** _____

**BALANCE & FLEXIBILITY NOTES**

**NUTRITION NOTES** _____    **RATING** [ ]

_____

_____

_____

_____

**BY THE NUMBERS** **5,117**: Average daily step count of Americans. **7,168**: Steps taken by Japanese. **9,695**: Steps taken by Western Australians. **18,425**: Steps taken by Amish men.

# TUESDAY

MORNING INFO

DAILY RATING

**CARDIO EXERCISE**

**TIME/DISTANCE/INTENSITY**

Cardio Notes

**STRENGTH TRAINING**

| | Weight | Reps | Weight | Reps | Weight | Reps |
|---|---|---|---|---|---|---|
| | | | | | | |
| | | | | | | |
| | | | | | | |
| | | | | | | |
| | | | | | | |
| | | | | | | |
| | | | | | | |
| | | | | | | |
| | | | | | | |
| | | | | | | |

Strength Notes

**BALANCE & FLEXIBILITY NOTES**

**NUTRITION NOTES**      RATING

**FITNESS FACTOID** The gluteus maximus is the body's largest muscle, but the masseter, a jaw muscle, is the strongest based on its weight. The soleus, a calf muscle, can pull with the greatest force.

# WEDNESDAY

MORNING INFO

DAILY RATING

**CARDIO EXERCISE**

**TIME/DISTANCE/INTENSITY**

**Cardio Notes**

| STRENGTH TRAINING | Weight | Reps | Weight | Reps | Weight | Reps |
|---|---|---|---|---|---|---|
| | | | | | | |
| | | | | | | |
| | | | | | | |
| | | | | | | |
| | | | | | | |
| | | | | | | |
| | | | | | | |
| | | | | | | |
| | | | | | | |
| | | | | | | |

**Strength Notes**

**BALANCE & FLEXIBILITY NOTES**

**NUTRITION NOTES**

RATING

**WEIGHT-CONTROL WISDOM** Losing 1.5 to 2 pounds a
week may be better long-term than slower weight loss, some research
suggests. Instant gratification — compliments, looser jeans, more
energy — may prove inspirational.

# THURSDAY

MORNING
INFO

DAILY
RATING

**CARDIO EXERCISE**

**TIME/DISTANCE/INTENSITY**

Cardio Notes

**STRENGTH TRAINING**

| | Weight | Reps | Weight | Reps | Weight | Reps |
|---|---|---|---|---|---|---|
| | | | | | | |
| | | | | | | |
| | | | | | | |
| | | | | | | |
| | | | | | | |
| | | | | | | |
| | | | | | | |
| | | | | | | |
| | | | | | | |
| | | | | | | |

Strength Notes

**BALANCE & FLEXIBILITY NOTES**

**NUTRITION NOTES**

RATING

**WORKOUT PAYOFF** Exercising in nature lowers mental-illness risk and improves your energy and sense of well-being, research shows. Even 5 minutes of "green exercise" can do the trick.

# FRIDAY

MORNING INFO [ ]

DAILY RATING [ ]

**CARDIO EXERCISE**

**TIME/DISTANCE/INTENSITY**

Cardio Notes

| STRENGTH TRAINING | Weight | Reps | Weight | Reps | Weight | Reps |
|---|---|---|---|---|---|---|
| | | | | | | |
| | | | | | | |
| | | | | | | |
| | | | | | | |
| | | | | | | |
| | | | | | | |
| | | | | | | |
| | | | | | | |
| | | | | | | |
| | | | | | | |

Strength Notes

BALANCE & FLEXIBILITY NOTES

NUTRITION NOTES        RATING [ ]

**TRAINING TRIVIA** The first bike race, 1,200 meters long, is thought to have been held in 1868 in Paris and won by a Brit who rode a wooden bicycle with iron tires. The Tour de France debuted in 1903.

# SATURDAY

MORNING INFO

DAILY RATING

**CARDIO EXERCISE**

**TIME/DISTANCE/INTENSITY**

Cardio Notes

| STRENGTH TRAINING | Weight | Reps | Weight | Reps | Weight | Reps |
|---|---|---|---|---|---|---|
| | | | | | | |
| | | | | | | |
| | | | | | | |
| | | | | | | |
| | | | | | | |
| | | | | | | |
| | | | | | | |
| | | | | | | |
| | | | | | | |
| | | | | | | |
| | | | | | | |

Strength Notes

**BALANCE & FLEXIBILITY NOTES**

**NUTRITION NOTES**

RATING

**CALORIE COUNT** 490 = 1 slice Starbucks banana nut loaf <u>or</u>
2 medium bananas + 12 walnut halves + 2 Fig Newtons

# SUNDAY

MORNING INFO

DAILY RATING

**CARDIO EXERCISE**

**TIME/DISTANCE/INTENSITY**

Cardio Notes

| STRENGTH TRAINING | Weight | Reps | Weight | Reps | Weight | Reps |
|---|---|---|---|---|---|---|
| | | | | | | |
| | | | | | | |
| | | | | | | |
| | | | | | | |
| | | | | | | |
| | | | | | | |
| | | | | | | |
| | | | | | | |
| | | | | | | |
| | | | | | | |

Strength Notes

**BALANCE & FLEXIBILITY NOTES**

**NUTRITION NOTES**

RATING

"On frosty mornings I lie in bed and wonder, If I didn't get up to ride today, who would know? The answer: I would."
— Olympic cyclist **KRISTIN ARMSTRONG**

# WEEKLY WRAP-UP

**WEEKLY RATING**

**Goals:** MET _____ EXCEEDED _____ MAYBE NEXT WEEK _____

HIGHLIGHT OF THE WEEK _____

**CARDIO NOTES**    TOTAL WORKOUTS [ ]    MILES/ YARDS [ ]    TOTAL TIME [ ]

_____

_____

_____

_____

**STRENGTH NOTES**    TOTAL WORKOUTS [ ]

_____

_____

_____

_____

**BALANCE & FLEXIBILITY NOTES**

**NUTRITION NOTES**    WEEKLY RATING [ ]

_____

_____

TOTAL WORKOUTS [ ]

_____

**THOUGHTS ABOUT THE WEEK**

# WEEK 2

Dates _____

Goals _____

_____

## MONDAY

MORNING INFO [ ]    DAILY RATING [ ]

**CARDIO EXERCISE** _____    **TIME/DISTANCE/INTENSITY** _____

_____    _____

_____    _____

_____    _____

Cardio Notes _____

| STRENGTH TRAINING | Weight | Reps | Weight | Reps | Weight | Reps |
|---|---|---|---|---|---|---|
| _____ | | | | | | |
| _____ | | | | | | |
| _____ | | | | | | |
| _____ | | | | | | |
| _____ | | | | | | |
| _____ | | | | | | |
| _____ | | | | | | |
| _____ | | | | | | |
| _____ | | | | | | |

Strength Notes _____

**BALANCE & FLEXIBILITY NOTES**

**NUTRITION NOTES**    **RATING** [ ]

_____

_____

_____

_____

**BY THE NUMBERS** **53**: Percent of American cats considered overweight. **43**: Percent of dogs considered overweight. **67**: Percent of American adults considered overweight.

# TUESDAY

| | | |
|---|---|---|
| MORNING INFO | | DAILY RATING |

**CARDIO EXERCISE**                                    **TIME/DISTANCE/INTENSITY**

_____              _____

_____              _____

_____              _____

Cardio Notes _____

**STRENGTH TRAINING**

| | Weight | Reps | Weight | Reps | Weight | Reps |
|---|---|---|---|---|---|---|
| _____ | | | | | | |
| _____ | | | | | | |
| _____ | | | | | | |
| _____ | | | | | | |
| _____ | | | | | | |
| _____ | | | | | | |
| _____ | | | | | | |
| _____ | | | | | | |
| _____ | | | | | | |
| _____ | | | | | | |

Strength Notes _____

_____

**BALANCE & FLEXIBILITY NOTES**          **NUTRITION NOTES**          RATING [ ]

_____

_____

_____

_____

**FITNESS FACTOID** Listening to music can make exercise seem less intense and increase endurance, speed, and power. Most effective: fast music and tunes you really dig.

# WEDNESDAY

MORNING INFO

DAILY RATING

**CARDIO EXERCISE**

**TIME/DISTANCE/INTENSITY**

Cardio Notes

| STRENGTH TRAINING | Weight | Reps | Weight | Reps | Weight | Reps |
|---|---|---|---|---|---|---|
| | | | | | | |
| | | | | | | |
| | | | | | | |
| | | | | | | |
| | | | | | | |
| | | | | | | |
| | | | | | | |
| | | | | | | |
| | | | | | | |
| | | | | | | |

Strength Notes

**BALANCE & FLEXIBILITY NOTES**

**NUTRITION NOTES**

RATING

**WEIGHT-CONTROL WISDOM** Among adults who maintained a 30-pound weight loss for at least one year, nearly two-thirds reported watching 10 or fewer hours of weekly TV. American adults average 28 hours of weekly TV viewing.

# THURSDAY

MORNING INFO

DAILY RATING

**CARDIO EXERCISE**

**TIME/DISTANCE/INTENSITY**

Cardio Notes

**STRENGTH TRAINING**

| Weight | Reps | Weight | Reps | Weight | Reps |
|--------|------|--------|------|--------|------|
| | | | | | |
| | | | | | |
| | | | | | |
| | | | | | |
| | | | | | |
| | | | | | |
| | | | | | |
| | | | | | |
| | | | | | |
| | | | | | |

Strength Notes

**BALANCE & FLEXIBILITY NOTES**

**NUTRITION NOTES**

RATING

**WORKOUT PAYOFF** In an 8-week study, yoga novices became 13 to 35 percent more flexible, could stand on one leg for 17 seconds longer, and could do 6 more push-ups.

# FRIDAY

**MORNING INFO**

**DAILY RATING**

**CARDIO EXERCISE**

**TIME/DISTANCE/INTENSITY**

**Cardio Notes**

| STRENGTH TRAINING | Weight | Reps | Weight | Reps | Weight | Reps |
|---|---|---|---|---|---|---|
| | | | | | | |
| | | | | | | |
| | | | | | | |
| | | | | | | |
| | | | | | | |
| | | | | | | |
| | | | | | | |
| | | | | | | |
| | | | | | | |

**Strength Notes**

**BALANCE & FLEXIBILITY NOTES**

**NUTRITION NOTES**  **RATING**

**TRAINING TRIVIA** Women were first allowed into the Boston Marathon in 1972, into the Olympic marathon in 1984, and into Olympic weightlifting and pole-vaulting in 2000.

# SATURDAY

MORNING INFO

DAILY RATING

| CARDIO EXERCISE | TIME/DISTANCE/INTENSITY |
|---|---|
| | |
| | |
| | |

Cardio Notes

| STRENGTH TRAINING | Weight | Reps | Weight | Reps | Weight | Reps |
|---|---|---|---|---|---|---|
| | | | | | | |
| | | | | | | |
| | | | | | | |
| | | | | | | |
| | | | | | | |
| | | | | | | |
| | | | | | | |
| | | | | | | |
| | | | | | | |

Strength Notes

BALANCE & FLEXIBILITY NOTES

NUTRITION NOTES          RATING

**CALORIE COUNT** 1,660 = Cold Stone Creamery 25-oz Milk and Cookies milkshake <u>or</u> homemade vanilla shake (2 cups 1 percent milk + 1 cup ice cream) + 11 homemade chocolate-chip cookies

# SUNDAY

MORNING INFO

DAILY RATING

**CARDIO EXERCISE**

**TIME/DISTANCE/INTENSITY**

Cardio Notes

| STRENGTH TRAINING | Weight | Reps | Weight | Reps | Weight | Reps |
|---|---|---|---|---|---|---|
| | | | | | | |
| | | | | | | |
| | | | | | | |
| | | | | | | |
| | | | | | | |
| | | | | | | |
| | | | | | | |
| | | | | | | |
| | | | | | | |

Strength Notes

**BALANCE & FLEXIBILITY NOTES**

**NUTRITION NOTES**

RATING

"You've got to have goals in life or you wither away."
— **JON MENDES**, 90, New York City Marathon finisher

# WEEKLY WRAP-UP

WEEKLY
RATING

**Goals:** MET _____ EXCEEDED _____ MAYBE NEXT WEEK _____

**HIGHLIGHT OF THE WEEK** _____

**CARDIO NOTES**          TOTAL
                          WORKOUTS [ ]          MILES/
                                                YARDS [ ]          TOTAL
                                                                   TIME [ ]

_____

_____

_____

_____

**STRENGTH NOTES**          TOTAL
                            WORKOUTS [ ]

_____

_____

_____

_____

**BALANCE & FLEXIBILITY NOTES**

                                          **NUTRITION NOTES**          WEEKLY
                                                                       RATING [ ]

                                          _____

                                          _____

                          TOTAL           _____
                          WORKOUTS [ ]
                                          _____

**THOUGHTS ABOUT THE WEEK**

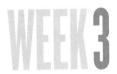 **WEEK 3**

Dates _____

Goals _____

_____

## MONDAY

MORNING INFO [ ]

DAILY RATING [ ]

**CARDIO EXERCISE** _____

**TIME/DISTANCE/INTENSITY** _____

_____  _____

_____  _____

_____  _____

**Cardio Notes** _____

| STRENGTH TRAINING | Weight | Reps | Weight | Reps | Weight | Reps |
|---|---|---|---|---|---|---|
| _____ | | | | | | |
| _____ | | | | | | |
| _____ | | | | | | |
| _____ | | | | | | |
| _____ | | | | | | |
| _____ | | | | | | |
| _____ | | | | | | |
| _____ | | | | | | |
| _____ | | | | | | |
| _____ | | | | | | |

**Strength Notes** _____

_____

**BALANCE & FLEXIBILITY NOTES**

**NUTRITION NOTES**     **RATING** [ ]

_____

_____

_____

_____

_____

# TUESDAY

MORNING INFO

DAILY RATING

**CARDIO EXERCISE**

**TIME/DISTANCE/INTENSITY**

Cardio Notes

**STRENGTH TRAINING**

| | Weight | Reps | Weight | Reps | Weight | Reps |
|---|---|---|---|---|---|---|
| | | | | | | |
| | | | | | | |
| | | | | | | |
| | | | | | | |
| | | | | | | |
| | | | | | | |
| | | | | | | |
| | | | | | | |
| | | | | | | |

Strength Notes

**BALANCE & FLEXIBILITY NOTES**

**NUTRITION NOTES**

RATING

**FITNESS FACTOID** Getting extra sleep improves athletic performance, alertness, and mood. After 8 weeks of sleeping 10 hours daily, football players' sprint times improved significantly.

# WEDNESDAY

MORNING INFO ☐     DAILY RATING ☐

**CARDIO EXERCISE**      **TIME/DISTANCE/INTENSITY**

_____    _____

_____    _____

_____    _____

Cardio Notes _____

| STRENGTH TRAINING | Weight | Reps | Weight | Reps | Weight | Reps |
|---|---|---|---|---|---|---|
| _____ | | | | | | |
| _____ | | | | | | |
| _____ | | | | | | |
| _____ | | | | | | |
| _____ | | | | | | |
| _____ | | | | | | |
| _____ | | | | | | |
| _____ | | | | | | |
| _____ | | | | | | |

Strength Notes _____

_____

**BALANCE & FLEXIBILITY NOTES**     **NUTRITION NOTES**    RATING ☐

_____

_____

_____

_____

_____

**WEIGHT-CONTROL WISDOM** When you slash calorie intake, your body compensates by moving less, so exercise is key for permanent weight loss.

# THURSDAY

MORNING INFO

DAILY RATING

**CARDIO EXERCISE**

**TIME/DISTANCE/INTENSITY**

Cardio Notes

| STRENGTH TRAINING | Weight | Reps | Weight | Reps | Weight | Reps |
|---|---|---|---|---|---|---|
| | | | | | | |
| | | | | | | |
| | | | | | | |
| | | | | | | |
| | | | | | | |
| | | | | | | |
| | | | | | | |
| | | | | | | |
| | | | | | | |
| | | | | | | |

Strength Notes

**BALANCE & FLEXIBILITY NOTES**

**NUTRITION NOTES**

RATING

**WORKOUT PAYOFF** People who exercise 7 hours a week have a **40** percent lower risk of dying prematurely than those active fewer than **30** minutes a week.

# FRIDAY

MORNING INFO

DAILY RATING

**CARDIO EXERCISE**

**TIME/DISTANCE/INTENSITY**

Cardio Notes

| STRENGTH TRAINING | Weight | Reps | Weight | Reps | Weight | Reps |
|---|---|---|---|---|---|---|
| | | | | | | |
| | | | | | | |
| | | | | | | |
| | | | | | | |
| | | | | | | |
| | | | | | | |
| | | | | | | |
| | | | | | | |
| | | | | | | |
| | | | | | | |

Strength Notes

**BALANCE & FLEXIBILITY NOTES**

**NUTRITION NOTES**

RATING

**TRAINING TRIVIA** Ancient Egyptians lifted heavy bags of sand as a form of exercise. Ancient Greeks lifted heavy stones.

# SATURDAY

| MORNING INFO | | DAILY RATING | |
| --- | --- | --- | --- |

**CARDIO EXERCISE**

**TIME/DISTANCE/INTENSITY**

**Cardio Notes**

**STRENGTH TRAINING**

| | Weight | Reps | Weight | Reps | Weight | Reps |
| --- | --- | --- | --- | --- | --- | --- |
| | | | | | | |
| | | | | | | |
| | | | | | | |
| | | | | | | |
| | | | | | | |
| | | | | | | |
| | | | | | | |
| | | | | | | |
| | | | | | | |
| | | | | | | |

**Strength Notes**

**BALANCE & FLEXIBILITY NOTES**

**NUTRITION NOTES**          **RATING**

**CALORIE COUNT** 530 = I Subway 6-inch tuna sub <u>or</u> I Subway 6-inch turkey sub + I apple + I tangerine + I package baby carrots + I stick string cheese

# SUNDAY

MORNING INFO

DAILY RATING

**CARDIO EXERCISE**

**TIME/DISTANCE/INTENSITY**

Cardio Notes

| STRENGTH TRAINING | Weight | Reps | Weight | Reps | Weight | Reps |
|---|---|---|---|---|---|---|
| | | | | | | |
| | | | | | | |
| | | | | | | |
| | | | | | | |
| | | | | | | |
| | | | | | | |
| | | | | | | |
| | | | | | | |
| | | | | | | |
| | | | | | | |

Strength Notes

**BALANCE & FLEXIBILITY NOTES**

**NUTRITION NOTES**

RATING

"Setbacks have an upside: They fuel new dreams."
— **DARA TORRES**, swimmer, five-time Olympian

# WEEKLY WRAP-UP

WEEKLY
RATING

**Goals:** MET _____ EXCEEDED _____ MAYBE NEXT WEEK _____

HIGHLIGHT OF THE WEEK _____

CARDIO NOTES      TOTAL WORKOUTS [ ]      MILES/ YARDS [ ]      TOTAL TIME [ ]

_____

_____

_____

_____

STRENGTH NOTES      TOTAL WORKOUTS [ ]

_____

_____

_____

_____

BALANCE & FLEXIBILITY NOTES

NUTRITION NOTES      WEEKLY RATING [ ]

_____

_____

TOTAL WORKOUTS [ ]

_____

THOUGHTS ABOUT THE WEEK

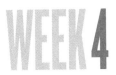

# WEEK 4

**Dates** _____

**Goals** _____
_____

## MONDAY

**MORNING INFO** ☐  **DAILY RATING** ☐

**CARDIO EXERCISE** _____

**TIME/DISTANCE/INTENSITY** _____

_____     _____

_____     _____

_____     _____

**Cardio Notes** _____

| STRENGTH TRAINING | Weight | Reps | Weight | Reps | Weight | Reps |
|---|---|---|---|---|---|---|
| _____ | | | | | | |
| _____ | | | | | | |
| _____ | | | | | | |
| _____ | | | | | | |
| _____ | | | | | | |
| _____ | | | | | | |
| _____ | | | | | | |
| _____ | | | | | | |
| _____ | | | | | | |
| _____ | | | | | | |

**Strength Notes** _____

**BALANCE & FLEXIBILITY NOTES**

**NUTRITION NOTES**     **RATING** ☐

_____

_____

_____

_____

**BY THE NUMBERS** **37**: Women's world record for pull-ups in 1 minute. **50**: Men's record. **67**: Women's record for pull-ups in 3 minutes. **100**: Men's 3-minute record.

# TUESDAY

MORNING INFO

DAILY RATING

**CARDIO EXERCISE**

**TIME/DISTANCE/INTENSITY**

Cardio Notes

| STRENGTH TRAINING | Weight | Reps | Weight | Reps | Weight | Reps |
|---|---|---|---|---|---|---|
| | | | | | | |
| | | | | | | |
| | | | | | | |
| | | | | | | |
| | | | | | | |
| | | | | | | |
| | | | | | | |
| | | | | | | |
| | | | | | | |
| | | | | | | |

Strength Notes

**BALANCE & FLEXIBILITY NOTES**

**NUTRITION NOTES**

RATING

**FITNESS FACTOID** Among world-class runners, average training pace is more strongly linked to marathon times than total miles run. Those who trained faster on fewer miles raced faster.

# WEDNESDAY

MORNING INFO

DAILY RATING

CARDIO EXERCISE

TIME/DISTANCE/INTENSITY

Cardio Notes

| STRENGTH TRAINING | Weight | Reps | Weight | Reps | Weight | Reps |
|---|---|---|---|---|---|---|
| | | | | | | |
| | | | | | | |
| | | | | | | |
| | | | | | | |
| | | | | | | |
| | | | | | | |
| | | | | | | |
| | | | | | | |
| | | | | | | |
| | | | | | | |

Strength Notes

BALANCE & FLEXIBILITY NOTES

NUTRITION NOTES

RATING

**WEIGHT-CONTROL WISDOM** Minor activity boosts, like standing instead of sitting, can boost calorie burn by 20 percent. Elevators, remotes, snowblowers, and other "conveniences" have cut daily energy burn by 100 to 200 calories.

# THURSDAY

MORNING INFO

DAILY RATING

CARDIO EXERCISE

TIME/DISTANCE/INTENSITY

_____

_____

_____

**Cardio Notes**

| STRENGTH TRAINING | Weight | Reps | Weight | Reps | Weight | Reps |
|---|---|---|---|---|---|---|
| _____ | | | | | | |
| _____ | | | | | | |
| _____ | | | | | | |
| _____ | | | | | | |
| _____ | | | | | | |
| _____ | | | | | | |
| _____ | | | | | | |
| _____ | | | | | | |
| _____ | | | | | | |

**Strength Notes**

**BALANCE & FLEXIBILITY NOTES**

NUTRITION NOTES          RATING

**WORKOUT PAYOFF** A 20-minute kettlebell workout can burn a gut-busting 20 calories per minute, equal to running a 6-minute mile or cross-country skiing uphill at a killer pace.

# FRIDAY

MORNING INFO

DAILY RATING

CARDIO EXERCISE

TIME/DISTANCE/INTENSITY

Cardio Notes

| STRENGTH TRAINING | Weight | Reps | Weight | Reps | Weight | Reps |
|---|---|---|---|---|---|---|
| | | | | | | |
| | | | | | | |
| | | | | | | |
| | | | | | | |
| | | | | | | |
| | | | | | | |
| | | | | | | |
| | | | | | | |
| | | | | | | |

Strength Notes

BALANCE & FLEXIBILITY NOTES

NUTRITION NOTES

RATING

**TRAINING TRIVIA** The word <u>dumbbell</u> originated in 15th-century England, when athletes would lift church bells with the clappers removed, making the bells "dumb," or silent.

# SATURDAY

MORNING INFO [ ]     DAILY RATING [ ]

**CARDIO EXERCISE**                    **TIME/DISTANCE/INTENSITY**

_____   _____
_____   _____
_____   _____

**Cardio Notes**
_____

| STRENGTH TRAINING | Weight | Reps | Weight | Reps | Weight | Reps |
|---|---|---|---|---|---|---|
| | | | | | | |
| | | | | | | |
| | | | | | | |
| | | | | | | |
| | | | | | | |
| | | | | | | |
| | | | | | | |
| | | | | | | |
| | | | | | | |

**Strength Notes**
_____

**BALANCE & FLEXIBILITY NOTES**        **NUTRITION NOTES**        RATING [ ]

_____
_____
_____
_____

**CALORIE COUNT** 470 = I Dunkin' Donuts wheat bagel + cream cheese <u>or</u> I slice whole-wheat toast + I tablespoon jam + 2 eggs + I cup strawberries + I cup plain nonfat yogurt

# SUNDAY

MORNING INFO

DAILY RATING

CARDIO EXERCISE

TIME/DISTANCE/INTENSITY

Cardio Notes

| STRENGTH TRAINING | Weight | Reps | Weight | Reps | Weight | Reps |
|---|---|---|---|---|---|---|
| | | | | | | |
| | | | | | | |
| | | | | | | |
| | | | | | | |
| | | | | | | |
| | | | | | | |
| | | | | | | |
| | | | | | | |
| | | | | | | |
| | | | | | | |

Strength Notes

BALANCE & FLEXIBILITY NOTES

NUTRITION NOTES

RATING

"I can't remember a single time I've felt worse after a run than before."
— **DEAN KARNAZES**, author of <u>Ultramarathon Man</u>

# WEEKLY WRAP-UP

WEEKLY
RATING [ ]

**Goals:** MET _____ EXCEEDED _____ MAYBE NEXT WEEK _____

HIGHLIGHT OF THE WEEK _____

CARDIO NOTES     TOTAL
WORKOUTS [ ]     MILES/
YARDS [ ]     TOTAL
TIME [ ]

_____
_____
_____
_____

STRENGTH NOTES     TOTAL
WORKOUTS [ ]

_____
_____
_____
_____

BALANCE & FLEXIBILITY NOTES

NUTRITION NOTES     WEEKLY
RATING [ ]

_____
_____

TOTAL
WORKOUTS [ ]

_____

THOUGHTS ABOUT THE WEEK

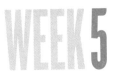 **WEEK 5**

Dates _____

Goals _____

_____

# MONDAY

MORNING INFO [ ]

DAILY RATING [ ]

**CARDIO EXERCISE** _____

**TIME/DISTANCE/INTENSITY** _____

_____    _____

_____    _____

_____    _____

**Cardio Notes** _____

| STRENGTH TRAINING | Weight | Reps | Weight | Reps | Weight | Reps |
|---|---|---|---|---|---|---|
| _____ | | | | | | |
| _____ | | | | | | |
| _____ | | | | | | |
| _____ | | | | | | |
| _____ | | | | | | |
| _____ | | | | | | |
| _____ | | | | | | |
| _____ | | | | | | |
| _____ | | | | | | |

**Strength Notes** _____

**BALANCE & FLEXIBILITY NOTES**

**NUTRITION NOTES** _____ **RATING** [ ]

_____

_____

_____

_____

# TUESDAY

MORNING INFO

DAILY RATING

**CARDIO EXERCISE**

**TIME/DISTANCE/INTENSITY**

Cardio Notes

| STRENGTH TRAINING | Weight | Reps | Weight | Reps | Weight | Reps |
|---|---|---|---|---|---|---|
| | | | | | | |
| | | | | | | |
| | | | | | | |
| | | | | | | |
| | | | | | | |
| | | | | | | |
| | | | | | | |
| | | | | | | |
| | | | | | | |

Strength Notes

**BALANCE & FLEXIBILITY NOTES**

**NUTRITION NOTES** RATING

**FITNESS FACTOID** The typical Tour de France rider's diet is 62 percent carbohydrate, 23 percent fat, and 15 percent protein.

# WEDNESDAY

MORNING INFO

DAILY RATING

**CARDIO EXERCISE**

**TIME/DISTANCE/INTENSITY**

**Cardio Notes**

| STRENGTH TRAINING | Weight | Reps | Weight | Reps | Weight | Reps |
|---|---|---|---|---|---|---|
| | | | | | | |
| | | | | | | |
| | | | | | | |
| | | | | | | |
| | | | | | | |
| | | | | | | |
| | | | | | | |
| | | | | | | |
| | | | | | | |
| | | | | | | |

**Strength Notes**

**BALANCE & FLEXIBILITY NOTES**

**NUTRITION NOTES**

**RATING**

**WEIGHT-CONTROL WISDOM** Tracking your every move with a pedometer or accelerometer is a proven way to boost activity. Setting a step or calorie-burn goal and recording daily totals helps too.

# THURSDAY

MORNING
INFO

DAILY
RATING

**CARDIO EXERCISE**

**TIME/DISTANCE/INTENSITY**

Cardio Notes

| STRENGTH TRAINING | Weight | Reps | Weight | Reps | Weight | Reps |
|---|---|---|---|---|---|---|
| | | | | | | |
| | | | | | | |
| | | | | | | |
| | | | | | | |
| | | | | | | |
| | | | | | | |
| | | | | | | |
| | | | | | | |
| | | | | | | |
| | | | | | | |

Strength Notes

**BALANCE & FLEXIBILITY NOTES**

**NUTRITION NOTES**          RATING

**WORKOUT PAYOFF** Insomniacs who exercised 40 minutes a day 4 days a week for 16 weeks reported better sleep quality and less daytime sleepiness, jumping from poor sleepers to good sleepers.

# FRIDAY

MORNING INFO

DAILY RATING

CARDIO EXERCISE

TIME/DISTANCE/INTENSITY

Cardio Notes

| STRENGTH TRAINING | Weight | Reps | Weight | Reps | Weight | Reps |
|---|---|---|---|---|---|---|

Strength Notes

BALANCE & FLEXIBILITY NOTES

NUTRITION NOTES

RATING

**TRAINING TRIVIA** The Mt. Everest Marathon, the planet's highest marathon, starts at 17,000 feet, near Everest Base Camp, and finishes at 11,300 feet. The record: 3:50:23.

# SATURDAY

| MORNING INFO | | DAILY RATING | |
|---|---|---|---|

**CARDIO EXERCISE**

**TIME/DISTANCE/INTENSITY**

_____

_____

_____

**Cardio Notes**

**STRENGTH TRAINING**

| | Weight | Reps | Weight | Reps | Weight | Reps |
|---|---|---|---|---|---|---|
| | | | | | | |
| | | | | | | |
| | | | | | | |
| | | | | | | |
| | | | | | | |
| | | | | | | |
| | | | | | | |
| | | | | | | |
| | | | | | | |

**Strength Notes**

**BALANCE & FLEXIBILITY NOTES**

**NUTRITION NOTES**    RATING

**CALORIE COUNT** 440 = I Burger King medium French fries <u>or</u> I medium baked sweet potato + 2 pats butter + I cup sautéed zucchini and onions

# SUNDAY

| MORNING INFO | | DAILY RATING | |

CARDIO EXERCISE _____  TIME/DISTANCE/INTENSITY _____

_____  _____

_____  _____

_____  _____

Cardio Notes _____

| STRENGTH TRAINING | Weight | Reps | Weight | Reps | Weight | Reps |
|---|---|---|---|---|---|---|
| _____ | | | | | | |
| _____ | | | | | | |
| _____ | | | | | | |
| _____ | | | | | | |
| _____ | | | | | | |
| _____ | | | | | | |
| _____ | | | | | | |
| _____ | | | | | | |
| _____ | | | | | | |

Strength Notes _____

_____

| BALANCE & FLEXIBILITY NOTES | NUTRITION NOTES | RATING | |
|---|---|---|---|

> "The whole idea of the finishing line was like reaching those Pearly Gates."
> — SISTER MADONNA BUDER, 76,
> oldest female Hawaii Ironman finisher

# WEEKLY WRAP-UP

WEEKLY RATING

**Goals:** MET _____ EXCEEDED _____ MAYBE NEXT WEEK _____

HIGHLIGHT OF THE WEEK _____

CARDIO NOTES     TOTAL WORKOUTS [ ]     MILES/ YARDS [ ]     TOTAL TIME [ ]

_____
_____
_____
_____
_____

STRENGTH NOTES     TOTAL WORKOUTS [ ]

_____
_____
_____
_____

BALANCE & FLEXIBILITY NOTES

NUTRITION NOTES     WEEKLY RATING [ ]

_____
_____
_____
_____

TOTAL WORKOUTS [ ]

THOUGHTS ABOUT THE WEEK

# WEEK 6

Dates _____

Goals _____
_____

## MONDAY

MORNING INFO [   ]     DAILY RATING [   ]

**CARDIO EXERCISE** _____     **TIME/DISTANCE/INTENSITY** _____

_____     _____

_____     _____

_____     _____

Cardio Notes _____

| STRENGTH TRAINING | Weight | Reps | Weight | Reps | Weight | Reps |
|---|---|---|---|---|---|---|
| _____ | | | | | | |
| _____ | | | | | | |
| _____ | | | | | | |
| _____ | | | | | | |
| _____ | | | | | | |
| _____ | | | | | | |
| _____ | | | | | | |
| _____ | | | | | | |
| _____ | | | | | | |

Strength Notes _____

**BALANCE & FLEXIBILITY NOTES**

**NUTRITION NOTES**     **RATING** [   ]

_____

_____

_____

_____

**BY THE NUMBERS** **1,576:** Steps climbed in the Empire State Building Run-Up. **86:** Flights of stairs. **9:33:** Men's record. **11:23:** Women's record. **22:15:** Time of 2011's oldest finisher, Ginette Bedard, age 77.

# TUESDAY

MORNING INFO

DAILY RATING

**CARDIO EXERCISE**

**TIME/DISTANCE/INTENSITY**

Cardio Notes

**STRENGTH TRAINING**

| Weight | Reps | Weight | Reps | Weight | Reps |
|--------|------|--------|------|--------|------|
|        |      |        |      |        |      |
|        |      |        |      |        |      |
|        |      |        |      |        |      |
|        |      |        |      |        |      |
|        |      |        |      |        |      |
|        |      |        |      |        |      |
|        |      |        |      |        |      |
|        |      |        |      |        |      |
|        |      |        |      |        |      |
|        |      |        |      |        |      |

Strength Notes

**BALANCE & FLEXIBILITY NOTES**

**NUTRITION NOTES**

RATING

**FITNESS FACTOID** The toughest sports — based on a combo of aerobic, strength, speed, power, flexibility, and agility — are triathlon, long jump, fencing, boxing, and tennis.

# WEDNESDAY

MORNING INFO ☐  DAILY RATING ☐

**CARDIO EXERCISE**

**TIME/DISTANCE/INTENSITY**

Cardio Notes

| STRENGTH TRAINING | Weight | Reps | Weight | Reps | Weight | Reps |
|---|---|---|---|---|---|---|
| | | | | | | |
| | | | | | | |
| | | | | | | |
| | | | | | | |
| | | | | | | |
| | | | | | | |
| | | | | | | |
| | | | | | | |
| | | | | | | |

Strength Notes

**BALANCE & FLEXIBILITY NOTES**

**NUTRITION NOTES**   RATING ☐

**WEIGHT-CONTROL WISDOM** Skipping meals lowers your metabolic rate and can cause muscle loss, so eat breakfast and every 3 to 5 hours after that.

# THURSDAY

MORNING INFO

DAILY RATING

**CARDIO EXERCISE**

**TIME/DISTANCE/INTENSITY**

Cardio Notes

| STRENGTH TRAINING | Weight | Reps | Weight | Reps | Weight | Reps |
|---|---|---|---|---|---|---|
|  |  |  |  |  |  |  |
|  |  |  |  |  |  |  |
|  |  |  |  |  |  |  |
|  |  |  |  |  |  |  |
|  |  |  |  |  |  |  |
|  |  |  |  |  |  |  |
|  |  |  |  |  |  |  |
|  |  |  |  |  |  |  |
|  |  |  |  |  |  |  |
|  |  |  |  |  |  |  |

Strength Notes

**BALANCE & FLEXIBILITY NOTES**

**NUTRITION NOTES**

RATING

**WORKOUT PAYOFF** Exercisers report fewer depression symptoms and less stress and anger than couch potatoes. Like anti-depressants, exercise affects neurotransmitter systems in the brain.

# FRIDAY

MORNING INFO

DAILY RATING

CARDIO EXERCISE

TIME/DISTANCE/INTENSITY

Cardio Notes

| STRENGTH TRAINING | Weight | Reps | Weight | Reps | Weight | Reps |
|---|---|---|---|---|---|---|
| | | | | | | |
| | | | | | | |
| | | | | | | |
| | | | | | | |
| | | | | | | |
| | | | | | | |
| | | | | | | |
| | | | | | | |
| | | | | | | |
| | | | | | | |

Strength Notes

BALANCE & FLEXIBILITY NOTES

NUTRITION NOTES

RATING

**TRAINING TRIVIA** The first triathlon — a 7k bike, 5k run, and 200m swim — was held in 1921 in France and called the Course Des Trois Sports. The first Ironman was held in 1978.

# SATURDAY

MORNING INFO

DAILY RATING

**CARDIO EXERCISE**

**TIME/DISTANCE/INTENSITY**

**Cardio Notes**

| STRENGTH TRAINING | Weight | Reps | Weight | Reps | Weight | Reps |
|---|---|---|---|---|---|---|
| | | | | | | |
| | | | | | | |
| | | | | | | |
| | | | | | | |
| | | | | | | |
| | | | | | | |
| | | | | | | |
| | | | | | | |
| | | | | | | |
| | | | | | | |

**Strength Notes**

**BALANCE & FLEXIBILITY NOTES**

**NUTRITION NOTES**          RATING

**CALORIE COUNT** 770 = I KFC Chicken Pot Pie <u>or</u> I Subway 6-inch Oven-Roasted Chicken sub + Tomato Garden Vegetable with Rotini soup + I apple

# SUNDAY

MORNING INFO

DAILY RATING

CARDIO EXERCISE

TIME/DISTANCE/INTENSITY

Cardio Notes

| STRENGTH TRAINING | Weight | Reps | Weight | Reps | Weight | Reps |
|---|---|---|---|---|---|---|
| | | | | | | |
| | | | | | | |
| | | | | | | |
| | | | | | | |
| | | | | | | |
| | | | | | | |
| | | | | | | |
| | | | | | | |
| | | | | | | |

Strength Notes

BALANCE & FLEXIBILITY NOTES

NUTRITION NOTES

RATING

"We all face adversity, but we all have two choices: give up or move on."
— **AMY PALMIERO-WINTERS**,
world-record amputee marathoner and triathlete

# WEEKLY WRAP-UP

WEEKLY
RATING ☐

**Goals:** MET _____ EXCEEDED _____ MAYBE NEXT WEEK _____

**HIGHLIGHT OF THE WEEK** _____

**CARDIO NOTES**    TOTAL WORKOUTS ☐    MILES/ YARDS ☐    TOTAL TIME ☐

_____

_____

_____

_____

**STRENGTH NOTES**    TOTAL WORKOUTS ☐

_____

_____

_____

_____

**BALANCE & FLEXIBILITY NOTES**

TOTAL WORKOUTS ☐

**NUTRITION NOTES**    WEEKLY RATING ☐

_____

_____

_____

_____

**THOUGHTS ABOUT THE WEEK**

# WEEK 7

Dates _____

Goals _____

_____

## MONDAY

MORNING INFO [        ]     DAILY RATING [    ]

**CARDIO EXERCISE** _____   **TIME/DISTANCE/INTENSITY** _____

_____   _____

_____   _____

_____   _____

**Cardio Notes** _____

| STRENGTH TRAINING | Weight | Reps | Weight | Reps | Weight | Reps |
|---|---|---|---|---|---|---|
| _____ | | | | | | |
| _____ | | | | | | |
| _____ | | | | | | |
| _____ | | | | | | |
| _____ | | | | | | |
| _____ | | | | | | |
| _____ | | | | | | |
| _____ | | | | | | |
| _____ | | | | | | |
| _____ | | | | | | |
| _____ | | | | | | |

**Strength Notes** _____

**BALANCE & FLEXIBILITY NOTES**

**NUTRITION NOTES**     **RATING** [    ]

_____

_____

_____

_____

**BY THE NUMBERS** **40 mph**: Top speed of a zebra. **35 mph**: Rabbit speed. **25 mph**: Elephant speed. **23.4 mph**: Top speed of male sprinters. **21.8**: Brown bear speed. **21.3 mph**: Top speed of women sprinters.

# TUESDAY

MORNING INFO

DAILY RATING

**CARDIO EXERCISE**

**TIME/DISTANCE/INTENSITY**

**Cardio Notes**

| STRENGTH TRAINING | Weight | Reps | Weight | Reps | Weight | Reps |
|---|---|---|---|---|---|---|
| | | | | | | |
| | | | | | | |
| | | | | | | |
| | | | | | | |
| | | | | | | |
| | | | | | | |
| | | | | | | |
| | | | | | | |
| | | | | | | |
| | | | | | | |

**Strength Notes**

**BALANCE & FLEXIBILITY NOTES**

**NUTRITION NOTES**

RATING

# WEDNESDAY

MORNING INFO

DAILY RATING

**CARDIO EXERCISE**

**TIME/DISTANCE/INTENSITY**

Cardio Notes

| STRENGTH TRAINING | Weight | Reps | Weight | Reps | Weight | Reps |
|---|---|---|---|---|---|---|
| | | | | | | |
| | | | | | | |
| | | | | | | |
| | | | | | | |
| | | | | | | |
| | | | | | | |
| | | | | | | |
| | | | | | | |
| | | | | | | |
| | | | | | | |
| | | | | | | |

Strength Notes

BALANCE & FLEXIBILITY NOTES

NUTRITION NOTES

RATING

**WEIGHT-CONTROL WISDOM** Women are more successful at slimming down when they add food-label reading to a workout program. Compare multiple products' calories, fiber, and saturated fat data before choosing.

# THURSDAY

MORNING INFO

DAILY RATING

**CARDIO EXERCISE**

**TIME/DISTANCE/INTENSITY**

Cardio Notes

| STRENGTH TRAINING | Weight | Reps | Weight | Reps | Weight | Reps |
|---|---|---|---|---|---|---|
| | | | | | | |
| | | | | | | |
| | | | | | | |
| | | | | | | |
| | | | | | | |
| | | | | | | |
| | | | | | | |
| | | | | | | |
| | | | | | | |
| | | | | | | |

Strength Notes

**BALANCE & FLEXIBILITY NOTES**

**NUTRITION NOTES**

RATING

**WORKOUT PAYOFF** Exercise reduces anxiety symptoms such as rapid breathing and a racing heart by 20 percent. Exercising 30 minutes or more works best.

# FRIDAY

MORNING INFO

DAILY RATING

CARDIO EXERCISE

TIME/DISTANCE/INTENSITY

Cardio Notes

| STRENGTH TRAINING | Weight | Reps | Weight | Reps | Weight | Reps |
|---|---|---|---|---|---|---|
| | | | | | | |
| | | | | | | |
| | | | | | | |
| | | | | | | |
| | | | | | | |
| | | | | | | |
| | | | | | | |
| | | | | | | |
| | | | | | | |
| | | | | | | |

Strength Notes

BALANCE & FLEXIBILITY NOTES

NUTRITION NOTES

RATING

**TRAINING TRIVIA** In the official sport of wife-carrying, men needn't carry their actual wives, but the women must weigh at least 49 kg (108 lbs). The track is 253.5 meters, with two dry obstacles and one water obstacle.

# SATURDAY

MORNING INFO

DAILY RATING

**CARDIO EXERCISE**

**TIME/DISTANCE/INTENSITY**

Cardio Notes

| STRENGTH TRAINING | Weight | Reps | Weight | Reps | Weight | Reps |
|---|---|---|---|---|---|---|
| | | | | | | |
| | | | | | | |
| | | | | | | |
| | | | | | | |
| | | | | | | |
| | | | | | | |
| | | | | | | |
| | | | | | | |
| | | | | | | |
| | | | | | | |

Strength Notes

**BALANCE & FLEXIBILITY NOTES**

**NUTRITION NOTES**   RATING

**CALORIE COUNT** 1,160 = 32-oz McDonald's Chocolate Triple Thick Shake <u>or</u> 12-oz McDonald's Chocolate Triple Thick Shake + double cheeseburger + small French fries + ketchup

# SUNDAY

MORNING INFO

DAILY RATING

**CARDIO EXERCISE**

**TIME/DISTANCE/INTENSITY**

Cardio Notes

| STRENGTH TRAINING | Weight | Reps | Weight | Reps | Weight | Reps |
|---|---|---|---|---|---|---|
| | | | | | | |
| | | | | | | |
| | | | | | | |
| | | | | | | |
| | | | | | | |
| | | | | | | |
| | | | | | | |
| | | | | | | |
| | | | | | | |
| | | | | | | |

Strength Notes

**BALANCE & FLEXIBILITY NOTES**

**NUTRITION NOTES**

RATING

"We didn't walk 2,200 miles, it's true, but here's the thing, we tried."
— BILL BRYSON, author, on attempting to hike the Appalachian Trail

# WEEKLY WRAP-UP

WEEKLY RATING ☐

**Goals:** MET _____ EXCEEDED _____ MAYBE NEXT WEEK _____

HIGHLIGHT OF THE WEEK _____

CARDIO NOTES          TOTAL WORKOUTS ☐          MILES/YARDS ☐          TOTAL TIME ☐

_____

_____

_____

_____

STRENGTH NOTES          TOTAL WORKOUTS ☐

_____

_____

_____

_____

BALANCE & FLEXIBILITY NOTES

NUTRITION NOTES          WEEKLY RATING ☐

_____

_____

_____

TOTAL WORKOUTS ☐

THOUGHTS ABOUT THE WEEK

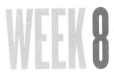WEEK 8

Dates _____

Goals _____

_____

## MONDAY

MORNING INFO [ ]

DAILY RATING [ ]

**CARDIO EXERCISE** _____

**TIME/DISTANCE/INTENSITY** _____

_____     _____

_____     _____

_____     _____

**Cardio Notes** _____

| STRENGTH TRAINING | Weight | Reps | Weight | Reps | Weight | Reps |
|---|---|---|---|---|---|---|
| | | | | | | |
| | | | | | | |
| | | | | | | |
| | | | | | | |
| | | | | | | |
| | | | | | | |
| | | | | | | |
| | | | | | | |
| | | | | | | |
| | | | | | | |

**Strength Notes** _____

**BALANCE & FLEXIBILITY NOTES**

**NUTRITION NOTES**     **RATING** [ ]

# TUESDAY

MORNING INFO

DAILY RATING

**CARDIO EXERCISE**

**TIME/DISTANCE/INTENSITY**

Cardio Notes

| STRENGTH TRAINING | Weight | Reps | Weight | Reps | Weight | Reps |
|---|---|---|---|---|---|---|
|  |  |  |  |  |  |  |
|  |  |  |  |  |  |  |
|  |  |  |  |  |  |  |
|  |  |  |  |  |  |  |
|  |  |  |  |  |  |  |
|  |  |  |  |  |  |  |
|  |  |  |  |  |  |  |
|  |  |  |  |  |  |  |
|  |  |  |  |  |  |  |
|  |  |  |  |  |  |  |

Strength Notes

**BALANCE & FLEXIBILITY NOTES**

**NUTRITION NOTES**          **RATING**

**FITNESS FACTOID** In 2000, for the first time in human history, the number of overweight adults surpassed those who are underweight.

# WEDNESDAY

MORNING INFO

DAILY RATING

| CARDIO EXERCISE | TIME/DISTANCE/INTENSITY |
|---|---|
| | |
| | |
| | |

Cardio Notes

| STRENGTH TRAINING | Weight | Reps | Weight | Reps | Weight | Reps |
|---|---|---|---|---|---|---|
| | | | | | | |
| | | | | | | |
| | | | | | | |
| | | | | | | |
| | | | | | | |
| | | | | | | |
| | | | | | | |
| | | | | | | |
| | | | | | | |
| | | | | | | |

Strength Notes

BALANCE & FLEXIBILITY NOTES

NUTRITION NOTES          RATING

**WEIGHT-CONTROL WISDOM** Interval training, alternating sprints with active recovery, may trigger more fat loss than continuous exercise, even when calorie burn is equal.

# THURSDAY

MORNING INFO

DAILY RATING

**CARDIO EXERCISE**

**TIME/DISTANCE/INTENSITY**

Cardio Notes

| STRENGTH TRAINING | Weight | Reps | Weight | Reps | Weight | Reps |
|---|---|---|---|---|---|---|
| | | | | | | |
| | | | | | | |
| | | | | | | |
| | | | | | | |
| | | | | | | |
| | | | | | | |
| | | | | | | |
| | | | | | | |
| | | | | | | |
| | | | | | | |
| | | | | | | |

Strength Notes

**BALANCE & FLEXIBILITY NOTES**

**NUTRITION NOTES** RATING

**WORKOUT PAYOFF** Exercising moms-to-be lower their risk of gestational diabetes and high blood pressure, and they're fitter and leaner 20 years after delivery than women inactive during pregnancy.

# FRIDAY

MORNING INFO ☐     DAILY RATING ☐

**CARDIO EXERCISE**

**TIME/DISTANCE/INTENSITY**

_____

_____

**Cardio Notes** _____

| STRENGTH TRAINING | Weight | Reps | Weight | Reps | Weight | Reps |
|---|---|---|---|---|---|---|
| _____ | | | | | | |
| _____ | | | | | | |
| _____ | | | | | | |
| _____ | | | | | | |
| _____ | | | | | | |
| _____ | | | | | | |
| _____ | | | | | | |
| _____ | | | | | | |
| _____ | | | | | | |

**Strength Notes** _____

**BALANCE & FLEXIBILITY NOTES**

**NUTRITION NOTES**     RATING ☐

**TRAINING TRIVIA** The sedentary lifestyle began circa 10,000 B.C., around the demise of the hunter-gatherer lifestyle, but didn't become a health problem until the 1950s, when we became ultra-slothful.

# SATURDAY

MORNING INFO

DAILY RATING

**CARDIO EXERCISE**

**TIME/DISTANCE/INTENSITY**

Cardio Notes

| STRENGTH TRAINING | Weight | Reps | Weight | Reps | Weight | Reps |
|---|---|---|---|---|---|---|
| | | | | | | |
| | | | | | | |
| | | | | | | |
| | | | | | | |
| | | | | | | |
| | | | | | | |
| | | | | | | |
| | | | | | | |
| | | | | | | |

Strength Notes

**BALANCE & FLEXIBILITY NOTES**

**NUTRITION NOTES**     RATING

**CALORIE COUNT** 1,200 = Large tub (20 cups) of popcorn at Regal Cinemas or 12 bags (72 cups) Orville Redenbacher's SmartPop! Gourmet Microwave Popcorn

# SUNDAY

MORNING INFO

DAILY RATING

**CARDIO EXERCISE**

**TIME/DISTANCE/INTENSITY**

Cardio Notes

| STRENGTH TRAINING | Weight | Reps | Weight | Reps | Weight | Reps |
|---|---|---|---|---|---|---|
| | | | | | | |
| | | | | | | |
| | | | | | | |
| | | | | | | |
| | | | | | | |
| | | | | | | |
| | | | | | | |
| | | | | | | |
| | | | | | | |
| | | | | | | |

Strength Notes

**BALANCE & FLEXIBILITY NOTES**

**NUTRITION NOTES**

RATING

"If you're not into it, just keep going and chances are the low feeling will pass."     — **PAM REED**, first person to run 300 miles without sleep

# WEEKLY WRAP-UP

WEEKLY RATING

**Goals:** MET _____ EXCEEDED _____ MAYBE NEXT WEEK _____

**HIGHLIGHT OF THE WEEK** _____

**CARDIO NOTES**     TOTAL WORKOUTS     MILES/ YARDS     TOTAL TIME

_____
_____
_____
_____

**STRENGTH NOTES**     TOTAL WORKOUTS

_____
_____
_____
_____

**BALANCE & FLEXIBILITY NOTES**

**NUTRITION NOTES**     WEEKLY RATING

_____
_____

TOTAL WORKOUTS

_____
_____

**THOUGHTS ABOUT THE WEEK**

# WEEK 9

**Dates** _____

**Goals** _____
_____

## MONDAY

**MORNING INFO** [ ]    **DAILY RATING** [ ]

**CARDIO EXERCISE** _____    **TIME/DISTANCE/INTENSITY** _____

_____    _____

_____    _____

_____    _____

**Cardio Notes** _____

| STRENGTH TRAINING | Weight | Reps | Weight | Reps | Weight | Reps |
|---|---|---|---|---|---|---|
| _____ | | | | | | |
| _____ | | | | | | |
| _____ | | | | | | |
| _____ | | | | | | |
| _____ | | | | | | |
| _____ | | | | | | |
| _____ | | | | | | |
| _____ | | | | | | |
| _____ | | | | | | |
| _____ | | | | | | |

**Strength Notes** _____

_____

**BALANCE & FLEXIBILITY NOTES**

**NUTRITION NOTES**    **RATING** [ ]

_____

_____

_____

_____

# TUESDAY

MORNING INFO

DAILY RATING

**CARDIO EXERCISE**

**TIME/DISTANCE/INTENSITY**

Cardio Notes

**STRENGTH TRAINING**

| | Weight | Reps | Weight | Reps | Weight | Reps |
|---|---|---|---|---|---|---|
| | | | | | | |
| | | | | | | |
| | | | | | | |
| | | | | | | |
| | | | | | | |
| | | | | | | |
| | | | | | | |
| | | | | | | |
| | | | | | | |
| | | | | | | |

Strength Notes

**BALANCE & FLEXIBILITY NOTES**

**NUTRITION NOTES**

RATING

**FITNESS FACTOID** Runners over age 40 need 1 to 3 days of rest or recovery workouts after a strenuous running session. Older runners should sub easy runs with cross-training activities.

# WEDNESDAY

MORNING INFO

DAILY RATING

CARDIO EXERCISE

TIME/DISTANCE/INTENSITY

Cardio Notes

| STRENGTH TRAINING | Weight | Reps | Weight | Reps | Weight | Reps |
|---|---|---|---|---|---|---|
| | | | | | | |
| | | | | | | |
| | | | | | | |
| | | | | | | |
| | | | | | | |
| | | | | | | |
| | | | | | | |
| | | | | | | |
| | | | | | | |
| | | | | | | |

Strength Notes

BALANCE & FLEXIBILITY NOTES

NUTRITION NOTES

RATING

**WEIGHT-CONTROL WISDOM** For each pound of muscle gained by weightlifting, you burn 5 to 10 extra calories per day — possibly enough to halt much of the nearly inevitable age-related weight gain.

# THURSDAY

MORNING INFO ☐

DAILY RATING ☐

**CARDIO EXERCISE**

**TIME/DISTANCE/INTENSITY**

Cardio Notes

| STRENGTH TRAINING | Weight | Reps | Weight | Reps | Weight | Reps |
|---|---|---|---|---|---|---|
| | | | | | | |
| | | | | | | |
| | | | | | | |
| | | | | | | |
| | | | | | | |
| | | | | | | |
| | | | | | | |
| | | | | | | |
| | | | | | | |

Strength Notes

**BALANCE & FLEXIBILITY NOTES**

**NUTRITION NOTES**

RATING ☐

**WORKOUT PAYOFF** Men with prostate cancer who exercised vigorously 3 or more hours a week had a 61 percent lower risk of dying from the disease compared to men who exercised less than 1 hour.

# FRIDAY

MORNING INFO

DAILY RATING

**CARDIO EXERCISE**

**TIME/DISTANCE/INTENSITY**

Cardio Notes

| STRENGTH TRAINING | Weight | Reps | Weight | Reps | Weight | Reps |
|---|---|---|---|---|---|---|
| | | | | | | |
| | | | | | | |
| | | | | | | |
| | | | | | | |
| | | | | | | |
| | | | | | | |
| | | | | | | |
| | | | | | | |
| | | | | | | |
| | | | | | | |
| | | | | | | |

Strength Notes

**BALANCE & FLEXIBILITY NOTES**

**NUTRITION NOTES**

RATING

**TRAINING TRIVIA** Yoga was developed 5,000 years ago by Hindu priests who imitated animal movements in hopes of achieving animal-like balance with nature.

# SATURDAY

MORNING INFO

DAILY RATING

**CARDIO EXERCISE**

**TIME/DISTANCE/INTENSITY**

**Cardio Notes**

| STRENGTH TRAINING | Weight | Reps | Weight | Reps | Weight | Reps |
|---|---|---|---|---|---|---|
| | | | | | | |
| | | | | | | |
| | | | | | | |
| | | | | | | |
| | | | | | | |
| | | | | | | |
| | | | | | | |
| | | | | | | |
| | | | | | | |
| | | | | | | |
| | | | | | | |

**Strength Notes**

**BALANCE & FLEXIBILITY NOTES**

**NUTRITION NOTES**          RATING

**CALORIE COUNT** 400 = 3.5-oz bag Raisinets <u>or</u> 3.5-oz bag
Gummi Bears + 3 cups grapes

# SUNDAY

MORNING INFO

DAILY RATING

**CARDIO EXERCISE**

**TIME/DISTANCE/INTENSITY**

Cardio Notes

| STRENGTH TRAINING | Weight | Reps | Weight | Reps | Weight | Reps |
|---|---|---|---|---|---|---|
| | | | | | | |
| | | | | | | |
| | | | | | | |
| | | | | | | |
| | | | | | | |
| | | | | | | |
| | | | | | | |
| | | | | | | |
| | | | | | | |
| | | | | | | |

Strength Notes

BALANCE & FLEXIBILITY NOTES

NUTRITION NOTES

RATING

"Try something new, even if you're not good at it."
— **LYNNE COX**, legendary cold-water distance swimmer

# WEEKLY WRAP-UP

**WEEKLY RATING** ☐

**Goals:**   MET _____   EXCEEDED _____   MAYBE NEXT WEEK _____

**HIGHLIGHT OF THE WEEK** _____

**CARDIO NOTES**   **TOTAL WORKOUTS** ☐   **MILES/ YARDS** ☐   **TOTAL TIME** ☐

_____
_____
_____
_____

**STRENGTH NOTES**   **TOTAL WORKOUTS** ☐

_____
_____
_____
_____

**BALANCE & FLEXIBILITY NOTES**

**NUTRITION NOTES**   **WEEKLY RATING** ☐

**TOTAL WORKOUTS** ☐

**THOUGHTS ABOUT THE WEEK**

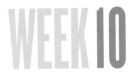 # WEEK 10

**Dates** _____

**Goals** _____
_____

## MONDAY

| MORNING INFO | | DAILY RATING | |
|---|---|---|---|

**CARDIO EXERCISE** _____

**TIME/DISTANCE/INTENSITY** _____

_____  _____

_____  _____

_____  _____

**Cardio Notes** _____

**STRENGTH TRAINING** _____

| Weight | Reps | Weight | Reps | Weight | Reps |
|---|---|---|---|---|---|

**Strength Notes** _____

**BALANCE & FLEXIBILITY NOTES**

**NUTRITION NOTES** _____ **RATING** [ ]

**BY THE NUMBERS** **38**: Age of oldest female Olympic marathon winner, Romania's Constantina Dita, in 2008. **37**: Age of oldest men's Olympic marathon winner, Portugal's Carlos Lopes, in 1984.

# TUESDAY

MORNING
INFO

DAILY
RATING

**CARDIO EXERCISE**

**TIME/DISTANCE/INTENSITY**

**Cardio Notes**

| STRENGTH TRAINING | Weight | Reps | Weight | Reps | Weight | Reps |
|---|---|---|---|---|---|---|
| | | | | | | |
| | | | | | | |
| | | | | | | |
| | | | | | | |
| | | | | | | |
| | | | | | | |
| | | | | | | |
| | | | | | | |
| | | | | | | |
| | | | | | | |

**Strength Notes**

**BALANCE & FLEXIBILITY NOTES**

**NUTRITION NOTES**         RATING

**FITNESS FACTOID** Walking uphill can burn 25 to 40 percent more calories than walking on flat ground, depending on the grade.

# WEDNESDAY

MORNING INFO

DAILY RATING

| CARDIO EXERCISE | TIME/DISTANCE/INTENSITY |
|---|---|
| | |
| | |
| | |

Cardio Notes

| STRENGTH TRAINING | Weight | Reps | Weight | Reps | Weight | Reps |
|---|---|---|---|---|---|---|
| | | | | | | |
| | | | | | | |
| | | | | | | |
| | | | | | | |
| | | | | | | |
| | | | | | | |
| | | | | | | |
| | | | | | | |
| | | | | | | |
| | | | | | | |

Strength Notes

BALANCE & FLEXIBILITY NOTES

NUTRITION NOTES

RATING

**WEIGHT-CONTROL WISDOM** On average, vegans are leaner than vegetarians, who are leaner than meat-eaters. Vegans eat fewer calories and more fiber, and the body seems to use plant calories more efficiently for fuel.

# THURSDAY

MORNING INFO

DAILY RATING

**CARDIO EXERCISE**

**TIME/DISTANCE/INTENSITY**

Cardio Notes

| STRENGTH TRAINING | Weight | Reps | Weight | Reps | Weight | Reps |
|---|---|---|---|---|---|---|
| | | | | | | |
| | | | | | | |
| | | | | | | |
| | | | | | | |
| | | | | | | |
| | | | | | | |
| | | | | | | |
| | | | | | | |
| | | | | | | |
| | | | | | | |

Strength Notes

**BALANCE & FLEXIBILITY NOTES**

**NUTRITION NOTES**          RATING

**WORKOUT PAYOFF** Moderate exercise boosts immunity.
In a 15-week study, women who walked 45 minutes a day 5 days a week
experienced fewer than half the sick days of women who didn't exercise.

# FRIDAY

MORNING INFO

DAILY RATING

CARDIO EXERCISE

TIME/DISTANCE/INTENSITY

Cardio Notes

| STRENGTH TRAINING | Weight | Reps | Weight | Reps | Weight | Reps |
|---|---|---|---|---|---|---|
| | | | | | | |
| | | | | | | |
| | | | | | | |
| | | | | | | |
| | | | | | | |
| | | | | | | |
| | | | | | | |
| | | | | | | |
| | | | | | | |

Strength Notes

BALANCE & FLEXIBILITY NOTES

NUTRITION NOTES

RATING

**TRAINING TRIVIA** Contrary to myth, the jumping jack was not invented by Jack LaLanne but apparently by John "Black Jack" Pershing, a hardboiled World War I general.

# SATURDAY

MORNING INFO ☐   DAILY RATING ☐

**CARDIO EXERCISE**                          **TIME/DISTANCE/INTENSITY**

_____                      _____
_____                      _____
_____                      _____

**Cardio Notes** _____

| STRENGTH TRAINING | Weight | Reps | Weight | Reps | Weight | Reps |
|---|---|---|---|---|---|---|
| _____ | | | | | | |
| _____ | | | | | | |
| _____ | | | | | | |
| _____ | | | | | | |
| _____ | | | | | | |
| _____ | | | | | | |
| _____ | | | | | | |
| _____ | | | | | | |
| _____ | | | | | | |

**Strength Notes** _____

**BALANCE & FLEXIBILITY NOTES**

**NUTRITION NOTES**        RATING ☐

_____
_____
_____
_____

**CALORIE COUNT** 1,300 = Dairy Queen Large Chocolate Malt or
12 Hershey's Kisses + 1 cup chocolate ice cream + 7 cups grapes

# SUNDAY

MORNING INFO

DAILY RATING

**CARDIO EXERCISE**

**TIME/DISTANCE/INTENSITY**

Cardio Notes

| STRENGTH TRAINING | Weight | Reps | Weight | Reps | Weight | Reps |
|---|---|---|---|---|---|---|
| | | | | | | |
| | | | | | | |
| | | | | | | |
| | | | | | | |
| | | | | | | |
| | | | | | | |
| | | | | | | |
| | | | | | | |
| | | | | | | |
| | | | | | | |

Strength Notes

BALANCE & FLEXIBILITY NOTES

NUTRITION NOTES

RATING

"I love that sense of satisfaction you get throughout the whole day knowing you've done your training session."

— **MELISSA MOON**, champion stairclimber

# WEEKLY WRAP-UP

WEEKLY RATING [ ]

**Goals:** MET _____ EXCEEDED _____ MAYBE NEXT WEEK _____

HIGHLIGHT OF THE WEEK _____

**CARDIO NOTES**     TOTAL WORKOUTS [ ]    MILES/ YARDS [ ]    TOTAL TIME [ ]

_____
_____
_____
_____

**STRENGTH NOTES**     TOTAL WORKOUTS [ ]

_____
_____
_____
_____

**BALANCE & FLEXIBILITY NOTES**

TOTAL WORKOUTS [ ]

**NUTRITION NOTES**    WEEKLY RATING [ ]

_____
_____
_____
_____

**THOUGHTS ABOUT THE WEEK**

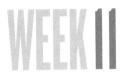
WEEK 11

Dates _____

Goals _____

_____

## MONDAY

MORNING INFO [          ]   DAILY RATING [    ]

**CARDIO EXERCISE** _____

**TIME/DISTANCE/INTENSITY** _____

_____   _____

_____   _____

_____   _____

**Cardio Notes** _____

| STRENGTH TRAINING | Weight | Reps | Weight | Reps | Weight | Reps |
|---|---|---|---|---|---|---|
| _____ | | | | | | |
| _____ | | | | | | |
| _____ | | | | | | |
| _____ | | | | | | |
| _____ | | | | | | |
| _____ | | | | | | |
| _____ | | | | | | |
| _____ | | | | | | |
| _____ | | | | | | |
| _____ | | | | | | |

**Strength Notes** _____

**BALANCE & FLEXIBILITY NOTES**

**NUTRITION NOTES**   **RATING** [    ]

_____

_____

_____

_____

**BY THE NUMBERS** **18,904**: Average daily steps taken by U.S. mail carriers. **12,991**: Steps taken by custodians. **10,087**: Steps taken by waiters. **5,062**: Steps taken by lawyers. **4,327**: Steps taken by secretaries.

# TUESDAY

MORNING INFO

DAILY RATING

### CARDIO EXERCISE

### TIME/DISTANCE/INTENSITY

**Cardio Notes**

### STRENGTH TRAINING

| | Weight | Reps | Weight | Reps | Weight | Reps |
|---|---|---|---|---|---|---|
| | | | | | | |

**Strength Notes**

**BALANCE & FLEXIBILITY NOTES**

**NUTRITION NOTES**

RATING

**FITNESS FACTOID** Exercise boosts math scores of overweight, inactive kids. Children who spent 40 minutes a day jump roping, hula hooping, and playing running games did better than kids who exercised for 20 minutes.

# WEDNESDAY

MORNING INFO

DAILY RATING

**CARDIO EXERCISE**

**TIME/DISTANCE/INTENSITY**

Cardio Notes

| STRENGTH TRAINING | Weight | Reps | Weight | Reps | Weight | Reps |
|---|---|---|---|---|---|---|
| | | | | | | |
| | | | | | | |
| | | | | | | |
| | | | | | | |
| | | | | | | |
| | | | | | | |
| | | | | | | |
| | | | | | | |
| | | | | | | |

Strength Notes

**BALANCE & FLEXIBILITY NOTES**

**NUTRITION NOTES**    RATING

# THURSDAY

MORNING INFO ☐       DAILY RATING ☐

**CARDIO EXERCISE**                    TIME/DISTANCE/INTENSITY

_____        _____

_____        _____

_____        _____

Cardio Notes _____

**STRENGTH TRAINING**

| | Weight | Reps | Weight | Reps | Weight | Reps |
|---|---|---|---|---|---|---|
| _____ | | | | | | |
| _____ | | | | | | |
| _____ | | | | | | |
| _____ | | | | | | |
| _____ | | | | | | |
| _____ | | | | | | |
| _____ | | | | | | |
| _____ | | | | | | |
| _____ | | | | | | |
| _____ | | | | | | |

Strength Notes _____

_____

**BALANCE & FLEXIBILITY NOTES**

NUTRITION NOTES        RATING ☐

_____

_____

_____

_____

**WORKOUT PAYOFF** Women with stronger quadriceps are less likely to get painful knee arthritis. For arthritis patients, regular exercise can ease pain.

# FRIDAY

MORNING INFO

DAILY RATING

**CARDIO EXERCISE**

**TIME/DISTANCE/INTENSITY**

Cardio Notes

| STRENGTH TRAINING | Weight | Reps | Weight | Reps | Weight | Reps |
|---|---|---|---|---|---|---|
| | | | | | | |
| | | | | | | |
| | | | | | | |
| | | | | | | |
| | | | | | | |
| | | | | | | |
| | | | | | | |
| | | | | | | |
| | | | | | | |
| | | | | | | |

Strength Notes

**BALANCE & FLEXIBILITY NOTES**

**NUTRITION NOTES**

RATING

**TRAINING TRIVIA** In a 1960 <u>Sports Illustrated</u> article titled "The Soft American," John F. Kennedy wrote, "We are under-exercised as a nation; we look instead of play; we ride instead of walk."

# SATURDAY

MORNING INFO

DAILY RATING

**CARDIO EXERCISE**

**TIME/DISTANCE/INTENSITY**

Cardio Notes

| STRENGTH TRAINING | Weight | Reps | Weight | Reps | Weight | Reps |
|---|---|---|---|---|---|---|
| | | | | | | |
| | | | | | | |
| | | | | | | |
| | | | | | | |
| | | | | | | |
| | | | | | | |
| | | | | | | |
| | | | | | | |
| | | | | | | |
| | | | | | | |

Strength Notes

**BALANCE & FLEXIBILITY NOTES**

**NUTRITION NOTES**          RATING

**CALORIE COUNT** 1,250 = Hardee's Double Thickburger <u>or</u> 8-oz New York strip steak + 1 baked potato + 2 pats butter + 1 cup green beans + 1 cup vanilla ice cream

# SUNDAY

MORNING INFO

DAILY RATING

**CARDIO EXERCISE**

**TIME/DISTANCE/INTENSITY**

Cardio Notes

| STRENGTH TRAINING | Weight | Reps | Weight | Reps | Weight | Reps |
|---|---|---|---|---|---|---|
| | | | | | | |
| | | | | | | |
| | | | | | | |
| | | | | | | |
| | | | | | | |
| | | | | | | |
| | | | | | | |
| | | | | | | |
| | | | | | | |
| | | | | | | |

Strength Notes

**BALANCE & FLEXIBILITY NOTES**

**NUTRITION NOTES**

RATING

"Ask yourself: Is that my best? If yes, you are headed in a great direction."
— **ANDY SPARKS**, U.S. Olympic track cycling coach

# WEEKLY WRAP-UP   WEEKLY RATING [ ]

**Goals:** MET _____ EXCEEDED _____ MAYBE NEXT WEEK _____

HIGHLIGHT OF THE WEEK _____

CARDIO NOTES        TOTAL WORKOUTS [ ]        MILES/ YARDS [ ]        TOTAL TIME [ ]

_____

_____

_____

_____

STRENGTH NOTES        TOTAL WORKOUTS [ ]

_____

_____

_____

_____

BALANCE & FLEXIBILITY NOTES

NUTRITION NOTES        WEEKLY RATING [ ]

_____

_____

TOTAL WORKOUTS [ ]

_____

THOUGHTS ABOUT THE WEEK

# WEEK 12

Dates _____

Goals _____

_____

## MONDAY

MORNING INFO [ ]     DAILY RATING [ ]

**CARDIO EXERCISE**

**TIME/DISTANCE/INTENSITY**

_____  _____

_____  _____

_____  _____

**Cardio Notes** _____

| STRENGTH TRAINING | Weight | Reps | Weight | Reps | Weight | Reps |
|---|---|---|---|---|---|---|
| _____ | | | | | | |
| _____ | | | | | | |
| _____ | | | | | | |
| _____ | | | | | | |
| _____ | | | | | | |
| _____ | | | | | | |
| _____ | | | | | | |
| _____ | | | | | | |
| _____ | | | | | | |
| _____ | | | | | | |

**Strength Notes** _____

_____

**BALANCE & FLEXIBILITY NOTES**

**NUTRITION NOTES**     RATING [ ]

_____

_____

_____

_____

**BY THE NUMBERS** **4:43.7**: Per-mile pace of Haile Gebrselassie while setting men's marathon record, 2:03:59. **5:10**: Pace of Paula Radcliffe while setting women's record, 2:15:25. **7:12**: Pace of the 1896 Olympic marathon winner.

# TUESDAY

MORNING INFO

DAILY RATING

**CARDIO EXERCISE**

**TIME/DISTANCE/INTENSITY**

Cardio Notes

**STRENGTH TRAINING**

| Weight | Reps | Weight | Reps | Weight | Reps |
|--------|------|--------|------|--------|------|
|        |      |        |      |        |      |
|        |      |        |      |        |      |
|        |      |        |      |        |      |
|        |      |        |      |        |      |
|        |      |        |      |        |      |
|        |      |        |      |        |      |
|        |      |        |      |        |      |
|        |      |        |      |        |      |
|        |      |        |      |        |      |
|        |      |        |      |        |      |

Strength Notes

**BALANCE & FLEXIBILITY NOTES**

**NUTRITION NOTES**    RATING

**FITNESS FACTOID** Walking poles can protect muscles and make hiking feel easier. When volunteers hiked 7 miles up and down, pole users reported less muscle pain and showed less strength loss days later.

# WEDNESDAY

MORNING INFO ☐  DAILY RATING ☐

**CARDIO EXERCISE** _____    **TIME/DISTANCE/INTENSITY** _____

_____    _____

_____    _____

**Cardio Notes** _____

| STRENGTH TRAINING | Weight | Reps | Weight | Reps | Weight | Reps |
|---|---|---|---|---|---|---|
| _____ | | | | | | |
| _____ | | | | | | |
| _____ | | | | | | |
| _____ | | | | | | |
| _____ | | | | | | |
| _____ | | | | | | |
| _____ | | | | | | |
| _____ | | | | | | |
| _____ | | | | | | |
| _____ | | | | | | |
| _____ | | | | | | |

**Strength Notes** _____

_____

**BALANCE & FLEXIBILITY NOTES**

**NUTRITION NOTES**    **RATING** ☐

_____

_____

_____

_____

**WEIGHT-CONTROL WISDOM** Financial stress contributes to weight gain, regardless of income. Over 9 years, obese women under the most financial stress gained 17 more pounds than those who could easily pay bills.

# THURSDAY

| MORNING INFO | | DAILY RATING | |

**CARDIO EXERCISE**

**TIME/DISTANCE/INTENSITY**

Cardio Notes

**STRENGTH TRAINING**

| Weight | Reps | Weight | Reps | Weight | Reps |
|--------|------|--------|------|--------|------|

Strength Notes

**BALANCE & FLEXIBILITY NOTES**

**NUTRITION NOTES**          RATING

**WORKOUT PAYOFF** Exercise reduces colon cancer risk by as much as **46 percent**. People who exercise consistently for at least 10 years have the lowest risk of colon cancer death.

# FRIDAY

MORNING INFO ☐          DAILY RATING ☐

**CARDIO EXERCISE**          TIME/DISTANCE/INTENSITY

Cardio Notes

| STRENGTH TRAINING | Weight | Reps | Weight | Reps | Weight | Reps |
|---|---|---|---|---|---|---|
| | | | | | | |
| | | | | | | |
| | | | | | | |
| | | | | | | |
| | | | | | | |
| | | | | | | |
| | | | | | | |
| | | | | | | |
| | | | | | | |

Strength Notes

**BALANCE & FLEXIBILITY NOTES**

NUTRITION NOTES          RATING ☐

**TRAINING TRIVIA** The 1950s medical establishment recommended pregnant women walk a max of one mile a day, broken up into several sessions.

# SATURDAY

| | MORNING INFO | | DAILY RATING | |

## CARDIO EXERCISE

### TIME/DISTANCE/INTENSITY

_____

_____

_____

**Cardio Notes**

## STRENGTH TRAINING

| STRENGTH TRAINING | Weight | Reps | Weight | Reps | Weight | Reps |
|---|---|---|---|---|---|---|
| | | | | | | |
| | | | | | | |
| | | | | | | |
| | | | | | | |
| | | | | | | |
| | | | | | | |
| | | | | | | |
| | | | | | | |

**Strength Notes**

**BALANCE & FLEXIBILITY NOTES**

**NUTRITION NOTES**        **RATING**

**CALORIE COUNT** 570 = Carl's Jr. Low Carb Six Dollar Burger <u>or</u> I hamburger patty (90 percent lean) + $1/2$ cup three-bean salad + $1/2$ cup cottage cheese + I cup pineapple + 4 Hershey's Kisses

# SUNDAY

MORNING INFO ☐

DAILY RATING ☐

**CARDIO EXERCISE**

TIME/DISTANCE/INTENSITY

_____ _____
_____ _____
_____ _____

Cardio Notes _____

**STRENGTH TRAINING**

| | Weight | Reps | Weight | Reps | Weight | Reps |
|---|---|---|---|---|---|---|
| _____ | | | | | | |
| _____ | | | | | | |
| _____ | | | | | | |
| _____ | | | | | | |
| _____ | | | | | | |
| _____ | | | | | | |
| _____ | | | | | | |
| _____ | | | | | | |
| _____ | | | | | | |
| _____ | | | | | | |

Strength Notes _____

**BALANCE & FLEXIBILITY NOTES**

NUTRITION NOTES

RATING ☐

_____
_____
_____
_____

"People ask me 'What was going through your mind in the race?' and I don't know."

— IAN THORPE, swimmer, five-time Olympic gold medalist

# WEEKLY WRAP-UP

WEEKLY RATING [ ]

**Goals:** MET _____ EXCEEDED _____ MAYBE NEXT WEEK _____

**HIGHLIGHT OF THE WEEK** _____

**CARDIO NOTES**    TOTAL WORKOUTS [ ]    MILES/ YARDS [ ]    TOTAL TIME [ ]

_____
_____
_____
_____

**STRENGTH NOTES**    TOTAL WORKOUTS [ ]

_____
_____
_____
_____

**BALANCE & FLEXIBILITY NOTES**

**NUTRITION NOTES**    WEEKLY RATING [ ]

_____
_____

TOTAL WORKOUTS [ ]

_____

**THOUGHTS ABOUT THE WEEK**

# WEEK 13

**Dates** _____

**Goals** _____

_____

## MONDAY

**MORNING INFO** ☐        **DAILY RATING** ☐

**CARDIO EXERCISE** _____        **TIME/DISTANCE/INTENSITY** _____

_____        _____

_____        _____

_____        _____

**Cardio Notes** _____

| STRENGTH TRAINING | Weight | Reps | Weight | Reps | Weight | Reps |
|---|---|---|---|---|---|---|
| _____ | | | | | | |
| _____ | | | | | | |
| _____ | | | | | | |
| _____ | | | | | | |
| _____ | | | | | | |
| _____ | | | | | | |
| _____ | | | | | | |
| _____ | | | | | | |
| _____ | | | | | | |
| _____ | | | | | | |

**Strength Notes** _____

**BALANCE & FLEXIBILITY NOTES**

**NUTRITION NOTES**        **RATING** ☐

_____

_____

_____

_____

# TUESDAY

| MORNING INFO | | DAILY RATING | |
|---|---|---|---|

**CARDIO EXERCISE**

**TIME/DISTANCE/INTENSITY**

_____   _____

_____   _____

_____   _____

**Cardio Notes**

_____

| STRENGTH TRAINING | Weight | Reps | Weight | Reps | Weight | Reps |
|---|---|---|---|---|---|---|
| _____ | | | | | | |
| _____ | | | | | | |
| _____ | | | | | | |
| _____ | | | | | | |
| _____ | | | | | | |
| _____ | | | | | | |
| _____ | | | | | | |
| _____ | | | | | | |
| _____ | | | | | | |

**Strength Notes**

_____

**BALANCE & FLEXIBILITY NOTES**

**NUTRITION NOTES**   **RATING** [ ]

_____

_____

_____

_____

**FITNESS FACTOID** Girls who walked or biked to school instead of getting a ride performed better in verbal and math tests, according to research on teens. An active commute lasting at least 15 minutes is best.

# WEDNESDAY

MORNING INFO

DAILY RATING

**CARDIO EXERCISE**

**TIME/DISTANCE/INTENSITY**

Cardio Notes

| STRENGTH TRAINING | Weight | Reps | Weight | Reps | Weight | Reps |
|---|---|---|---|---|---|---|
| | | | | | | |
| | | | | | | |
| | | | | | | |
| | | | | | | |
| | | | | | | |
| | | | | | | |
| | | | | | | |
| | | | | | | |
| | | | | | | |

Strength Notes

**BALANCE & FLEXIBILITY NOTES**

**NUTRITION NOTES**

RATING

**WEIGHT-CONTROL WISDOM** If you limit variety of foods and flavors — within a day, a meal, even a sandwich — you can achieve satisfaction before your calorie count skyrockets, research shows.

# THURSDAY

MORNING INFO

DAILY RATING

**CARDIO EXERCISE**

**TIME/DISTANCE/INTENSITY**

Cardio Notes

| STRENGTH TRAINING | Weight | Reps | Weight | Reps | Weight | Reps |
|---|---|---|---|---|---|---|
| | | | | | | |
| | | | | | | |
| | | | | | | |
| | | | | | | |
| | | | | | | |
| | | | | | | |
| | | | | | | |
| | | | | | | |
| | | | | | | |

Strength Notes

**BALANCE & FLEXIBILITY NOTES**

**NUTRITION NOTES**

RATING

**WORKOUT PAYOFF** Exercise lowers your risk of coronary heart disease, America's top killer, by as much as 50 percent. Sedentary folks have the same heart-disease risk as smokers.

# FRIDAY

MORNING INFO

DAILY RATING

| CARDIO EXERCISE | TIME/DISTANCE/INTENSITY |
|---|---|
| | |
| | |
| | |

Cardio Notes

| STRENGTH TRAINING | Weight | Reps | Weight | Reps | Weight | Reps |
|---|---|---|---|---|---|---|
| | | | | | | |
| | | | | | | |
| | | | | | | |
| | | | | | | |
| | | | | | | |
| | | | | | | |
| | | | | | | |
| | | | | | | |
| | | | | | | |

Strength Notes

BALANCE & FLEXIBILITY NOTES

NUTRITION NOTES          RATING

# SATURDAY

MORNING INFO

DAILY RATING

**CARDIO EXERCISE**

**TIME/DISTANCE/INTENSITY**

Cardio Notes

| STRENGTH TRAINING | Weight | Reps | Weight | Reps | Weight | Reps |
|---|---|---|---|---|---|---|
| | | | | | | |
| | | | | | | |
| | | | | | | |
| | | | | | | |
| | | | | | | |
| | | | | | | |
| | | | | | | |
| | | | | | | |
| | | | | | | |

Strength Notes

**BALANCE & FLEXIBILITY NOTES**

**NUTRITION NOTES**          RATING

**CALORIE COUNT** 800 = Taco Bell Fiesta Taco Salad <u>or</u>
9 1/2 slices medium Pizza Hut Veggie Edge Pizza

# SUNDAY

MORNING INFO ☐      DAILY RATING ☐

| CARDIO EXERCISE | TIME/DISTANCE/INTENSITY |
|---|---|
| _____ | _____ |
| _____ | _____ |
| _____ | _____ |

Cardio Notes _____

| STRENGTH TRAINING | Weight | Reps | Weight | Reps | Weight | Reps |
|---|---|---|---|---|---|---|
| _____ | | | | | | |
| _____ | | | | | | |
| _____ | | | | | | |
| _____ | | | | | | |
| _____ | | | | | | |
| _____ | | | | | | |
| _____ | | | | | | |
| _____ | | | | | | |
| _____ | | | | | | |
| _____ | | | | | | |

Strength Notes _____

BALANCE & FLEXIBILITY NOTES

NUTRITION NOTES      RATING ☐

"If you want to excel at anything, you have to have a plan."
— **JERZY GREGOREK**, world-champion weightlifter

# WEEKLY WRAP-UP

WEEKLY
RATING

**Goals:** MET _____ EXCEEDED _____ MAYBE NEXT WEEK _____

**HIGHLIGHT OF THE WEEK** _____

**CARDIO NOTES**    TOTAL WORKOUTS          MILES/ YARDS          TOTAL TIME

_____
_____
_____
_____

**STRENGTH NOTES**    TOTAL WORKOUTS

_____
_____
_____
_____

**BALANCE & FLEXIBILITY NOTES**

**NUTRITION NOTES**          WEEKLY RATING

_____

_____

TOTAL WORKOUTS          _____

**THOUGHTS ABOUT THE WEEK**

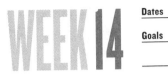
# WEEK 14

Dates _____

Goals _____

_____

## MONDAY

MORNING INFO [ ]    DAILY RATING [ ]

**CARDIO EXERCISE** _____    **TIME/DISTANCE/INTENSITY** _____

_____    _____

_____    _____

_____    _____

**Cardio Notes** _____

| STRENGTH TRAINING | Weight | Reps | Weight | Reps | Weight | Reps |
|---|---|---|---|---|---|---|
| _____ | | | | | | |
| _____ | | | | | | |
| _____ | | | | | | |
| _____ | | | | | | |
| _____ | | | | | | |
| _____ | | | | | | |
| _____ | | | | | | |
| _____ | | | | | | |
| _____ | | | | | | |
| _____ | | | | | | |
| _____ | | | | | | |

**Strength Notes** _____

**BALANCE & FLEXIBILITY NOTES**

**NUTRITION NOTES**     **RATING** [ ]

_____

_____

_____

_____

**BY THE NUMBERS** **3**: Hours per day that 9-year-olds are moderately physically active. **49**: Minutes per weekday that 15-year-olds are active. **35**: Minutes per weekend day that 15-year-olds are active.

# TUESDAY

MORNING INFO

DAILY RATING

**CARDIO EXERCISE**

**TIME/DISTANCE/INTENSITY**

Cardio Notes

**STRENGTH TRAINING**

| | Weight | Reps | Weight | Reps | Weight | Reps |
|---|---|---|---|---|---|---|

Strength Notes

**BALANCE & FLEXIBILITY NOTES**

**NUTRITION NOTES**

RATING

**FITNESS FACTOID** Even people with a strong genetic predisposition to obesity can offset their risk of being overweight by being physically active.

# WEDNESDAY

MORNING INFO

DAILY RATING

**CARDIO EXERCISE**

TIME/DISTANCE/INTENSITY

Cardio Notes

| STRENGTH TRAINING | Weight | Reps | Weight | Reps | Weight | Reps |
|---|---|---|---|---|---|---|
| | | | | | | |
| | | | | | | |
| | | | | | | |
| | | | | | | |
| | | | | | | |
| | | | | | | |
| | | | | | | |
| | | | | | | |
| | | | | | | |
| | | | | | | |

Strength Notes

**BALANCE & FLEXIBILITY NOTES**

**NUTRITION NOTES**

RATING

**WEIGHT-CONTROL WISDOM** Women who took smaller bites, chewed more, and put forks down between bites ate 10 percent fewer calories and felt more satisfied than when they ate quickly.

# THURSDAY

MORNING INFO

DAILY RATING

**CARDIO EXERCISE**

**TIME/DISTANCE/INTENSITY**

Cardio Notes

**STRENGTH TRAINING**

| | Weight | Reps | Weight | Reps | Weight | Reps |
|---|---|---|---|---|---|---|
| | | | | | | |

Strength Notes

**BALANCE & FLEXIBILITY NOTES**

**NUTRITION NOTES**

RATING

**WORKOUT PAYOFF** Exercisers have about a 30 percent lower risk of developing high blood pressure than couch potatoes.

# FRIDAY

MORNING INFO

DAILY RATING

**CARDIO EXERCISE**

**TIME/DISTANCE/INTENSITY**

Cardio Notes

| STRENGTH TRAINING | Weight | Reps | Weight | Reps | Weight | Reps |
|---|---|---|---|---|---|---|
| | | | | | | |
| | | | | | | |
| | | | | | | |
| | | | | | | |
| | | | | | | |
| | | | | | | |
| | | | | | | |
| | | | | | | |
| | | | | | | |
| | | | | | | |

Strength Notes

**BALANCE & FLEXIBILITY NOTES**

**NUTRITION NOTES**

RATING

**TRAINING TRIVIA** Doctors of the 1890s cautioned that competitive cyclists might develop a permanent grimace dubbed "bicycle face" and might damage their lungs due to the arched "monkey hump" position.

# SATURDAY

MORNING INFO

DAILY RATING

**CARDIO EXERCISE**

**TIME/DISTANCE/INTENSITY**

Cardio Notes

**STRENGTH TRAINING**

| | Weight | Reps | Weight | Reps | Weight | Reps |
|---|---|---|---|---|---|---|

Strength Notes

**BALANCE & FLEXIBILITY NOTES**

**NUTRITION NOTES**

RATING

## CALORIE COUNT 1,300 = Baja Fresh chips and guacamole or Chicken Bare Burrito (in a bowl, no tortilla) + tortilla soup

# SUNDAY

MORNING INFO

DAILY RATING

**CARDIO EXERCISE**

**TIME/DISTANCE/INTENSITY**

Cardio Notes

**STRENGTH TRAINING**

| Weight | Reps | Weight | Reps | Weight | Reps |
|--------|------|--------|------|--------|------|
|        |      |        |      |        |      |
|        |      |        |      |        |      |
|        |      |        |      |        |      |
|        |      |        |      |        |      |
|        |      |        |      |        |      |
|        |      |        |      |        |      |
|        |      |        |      |        |      |
|        |      |        |      |        |      |
|        |      |        |      |        |      |
|        |      |        |      |        |      |

Strength Notes

**BALANCE & FLEXIBILITY NOTES**

**NUTRITION NOTES**

RATING

"You can't put a limit on anything. The more you dream, the farther you get."
— **MICHAEL PHELPS**, swimmer, winner of 16 Olympic medals

# WEEKLY WRAP-UP

WEEKLY RATING [ ]

**Goals:** MET _____ EXCEEDED _____ MAYBE NEXT WEEK _____

HIGHLIGHT OF THE WEEK _____

CARDIO NOTES          TOTAL WORKOUTS [ ]      MILES/ YARDS [ ]          TOTAL TIME [ ]

_____

_____

_____

_____

STRENGTH NOTES          TOTAL WORKOUTS [ ]

_____

_____

_____

_____

BALANCE & FLEXIBILITY NOTES

NUTRITION NOTES          WEEKLY RATING [ ]

_____

_____

TOTAL WORKOUTS [ ]          _____

THOUGHTS ABOUT THE WEEK

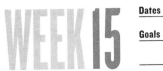WEEK 15

Dates _____

Goals _____

_____

## MONDAY

MORNING INFO [ ]   DAILY RATING [ ]

**CARDIO EXERCISE** _____

**TIME/DISTANCE/INTENSITY** _____

_____   _____

_____   _____

_____   _____

Cardio Notes _____

| STRENGTH TRAINING | Weight | Reps | Weight | Reps | Weight | Reps |
|---|---|---|---|---|---|---|
| _____ | | | | | | |
| _____ | | | | | | |
| _____ | | | | | | |
| _____ | | | | | | |
| _____ | | | | | | |
| _____ | | | | | | |
| _____ | | | | | | |
| _____ | | | | | | |
| _____ | | | | | | |
| _____ | | | | | | |

Strength Notes _____

**BALANCE & FLEXIBILITY NOTES**

**NUTRITION NOTES**     RATING [ ]

_____

_____

_____

_____

# TUESDAY

MORNING
INFO

DAILY
RATING

**CARDIO EXERCISE**

**TIME/DISTANCE/INTENSITY**

**Cardio Notes**

| STRENGTH TRAINING | Weight | Reps | Weight | Reps | Weight | Reps |
|---|---|---|---|---|---|---|
| | | | | | | |
| | | | | | | |
| | | | | | | |
| | | | | | | |
| | | | | | | |
| | | | | | | |
| | | | | | | |
| | | | | | | |
| | | | | | | |
| | | | | | | |

**Strength Notes**

**BALANCE & FLEXIBILITY NOTES**

**NUTRITION NOTES**          **RATING**

**FITNESS FACTOID** Even exercisers who spend most of the day sitting have an elevated cardiovascular disease risk. Television watching has been linked with greater risk for obesity and Type 2 diabetes.

# WEDNESDAY

MORNING INFO

DAILY RATING

| CARDIO EXERCISE | TIME/DISTANCE/INTENSITY |
|---|---|
| | |
| | |
| | |

Cardio Notes

| STRENGTH TRAINING | Weight | Reps | Weight | Reps | Weight | Reps |
|---|---|---|---|---|---|---|
| | | | | | | |
| | | | | | | |
| | | | | | | |
| | | | | | | |
| | | | | | | |
| | | | | | | |
| | | | | | | |
| | | | | | | |
| | | | | | | |

Strength Notes

BALANCE & FLEXIBILITY NOTES

NUTRITION NOTES          RATING

**WEIGHT-CONTROL WISDOM** To limit calories at a Chinese buffet, browse the food before serving yourself, use chopsticks and small plates, place a napkin on your lap, and sit facing away from the food.

# THURSDAY

MORNING INFO ☐    DAILY RATING ☐

**CARDIO EXERCISE**    **TIME/DISTANCE/INTENSITY**

_____    _____

_____    _____

_____    _____

**Cardio Notes** _____

**STRENGTH TRAINING**

| | Weight | Reps | Weight | Reps | Weight | Reps |
|---|---|---|---|---|---|---|
| | | | | | | |
| | | | | | | |
| | | | | | | |
| | | | | | | |
| | | | | | | |
| | | | | | | |
| | | | | | | |
| | | | | | | |
| | | | | | | |
| | | | | | | |

**Strength Notes** _____

**BALANCE & FLEXIBILITY NOTES**

**NUTRITION NOTES**    RATING ☐

_____

_____

_____

_____

_____

**WORKOUT PAYOFF** Lifting weights can halt, and maybe even reverse, the decline in bone mass that starts after age 30.

# FRIDAY

MORNING INFO

DAILY RATING

**CARDIO EXERCISE**

**TIME/DISTANCE/INTENSITY**

**Cardio Notes**

| STRENGTH TRAINING | Weight | Reps | Weight | Reps | Weight | Reps |
|---|---|---|---|---|---|---|
| | | | | | | |
| | | | | | | |
| | | | | | | |
| | | | | | | |
| | | | | | | |
| | | | | | | |
| | | | | | | |
| | | | | | | |
| | | | | | | |
| | | | | | | |

**Strength Notes**

**BALANCE & FLEXIBILITY NOTES**

**NUTRITION NOTES**

RATING

**TRAINING TRIVIA** Pole-vaulting was developed circa 1820 B.C. by the ancient Irish Celts, who likely used tree limbs to vault across streams.

# SATURDAY

MORNING INFO

DAILY RATING

**CARDIO EXERCISE**

**TIME/DISTANCE/INTENSITY**

Cardio Notes

| STRENGTH TRAINING | Weight | Reps | Weight | Reps | Weight | Reps |
|---|---|---|---|---|---|---|
| | | | | | | |
| | | | | | | |
| | | | | | | |
| | | | | | | |
| | | | | | | |
| | | | | | | |
| | | | | | | |
| | | | | | | |
| | | | | | | |
| | | | | | | |

Strength Notes

**BALANCE & FLEXIBILITY NOTES**

**NUTRITION NOTES**          RATING

**CALORIE COUNT** 780 = McDonald's Happy Meal with cheeseburger, fries, and milk <u>or</u> 2 Happy Meals with chicken nuggets, apple slices, and milk

# SUNDAY

MORNING INFO

DAILY RATING

**CARDIO EXERCISE**

**TIME/DISTANCE/INTENSITY**

Cardio Notes

| STRENGTH TRAINING | Weight | Reps | Weight | Reps | Weight | Reps |
|---|---|---|---|---|---|---|
| | | | | | | |
| | | | | | | |
| | | | | | | |
| | | | | | | |
| | | | | | | |
| | | | | | | |
| | | | | | | |
| | | | | | | |
| | | | | | | |

Strength Notes

**BALANCE & FLEXIBILITY NOTES**

**NUTRITION NOTES**

RATING

"Surround yourself with inspired and motivated people with similar high-minded goals."

— **SARAH HAMMER**, track cyclist, Olympian, and world champion

# WEEKLY WRAP-UP

WEEKLY RATING

**Goals:** MET _____ EXCEEDED _____ MAYBE NEXT WEEK _____

HIGHLIGHT OF THE WEEK _____

CARDIO NOTES     TOTAL WORKOUTS [ ]     MILES/YARDS [ ]     TOTAL TIME [ ]

_____

_____

_____

_____

STRENGTH NOTES     TOTAL WORKOUTS [ ]

_____

_____

_____

_____

BALANCE & FLEXIBILITY NOTES

NUTRITION NOTES     WEEKLY RATING [ ]

_____

_____

TOTAL WORKOUTS [ ]

_____

THOUGHTS ABOUT THE WEEK

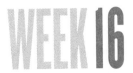
# WEEK 16

**Dates** _____

**Goals** _____
_____

## MONDAY

MORNING INFO [ ]     DAILY RATING [ ]

**CARDIO EXERCISE** _____     **TIME/DISTANCE/INTENSITY** _____

_____     _____

_____     _____

_____     _____

**Cardio Notes** _____

| STRENGTH TRAINING | Weight | Reps | Weight | Reps | Weight | Reps |
|---|---|---|---|---|---|---|
| _____ | | | | | | |
| _____ | | | | | | |
| _____ | | | | | | |
| _____ | | | | | | |
| _____ | | | | | | |
| _____ | | | | | | |
| _____ | | | | | | |
| _____ | | | | | | |
| _____ | | | | | | |
| _____ | | | | | | |

**Strength Notes** _____

**BALANCE & FLEXIBILITY NOTES**

**NUTRITION NOTES** _____     **RATING** [ ]

_____
_____
_____
_____

**BY THE NUMBERS** **6:25**: World record for walking one mile. **7:13**: Fastest mile walked on stilts. **12:23**: Fastest mile on non-spring-loaded stilts.

# TUESDAY

MORNING INFO

DAILY RATING

**CARDIO EXERCISE**

**TIME/DISTANCE/INTENSITY**

**Cardio Notes**

| STRENGTH TRAINING | Weight | Reps | Weight | Reps | Weight | Reps |
|---|---|---|---|---|---|---|
| | | | | | | |
| | | | | | | |
| | | | | | | |
| | | | | | | |
| | | | | | | |
| | | | | | | |
| | | | | | | |
| | | | | | | |
| | | | | | | |
| | | | | | | |
| | | | | | | |

**Strength Notes**

**BALANCE & FLEXIBILITY NOTES**

**NUTRITION NOTES**         RATING

**FITNESS FACTOID** Resistance training is likely to have a more pronounced effect on running distances less than 10k than it does on performance at distances beyond 10k.

# WEDNESDAY

MORNING INFO

DAILY RATING

| CARDIO EXERCISE | TIME/DISTANCE/INTENSITY |
|---|---|
| | |
| | |
| | |

Cardio Notes

| STRENGTH TRAINING | Weight | Reps | Weight | Reps | Weight | Reps |
|---|---|---|---|---|---|---|
| | | | | | | |
| | | | | | | |
| | | | | | | |
| | | | | | | |
| | | | | | | |
| | | | | | | |
| | | | | | | |
| | | | | | | |
| | | | | | | |
| | | | | | | |

Strength Notes

BALANCE & FLEXIBILITY NOTES

NUTRITION NOTES

RATING

**WEIGHT-CONTROL WISDOM** We eat roughly the same volume of food each day, so choose lower-calorie options that take up space, like puffed cereals and water-laden foods such as fruits, veggies, and soups.

# THURSDAY

MORNING INFO

DAILY RATING

**CARDIO EXERCISE**

**TIME/DISTANCE/INTENSITY**

Cardio Notes

| STRENGTH TRAINING | Weight | Reps | Weight | Reps | Weight | Reps |
|---|---|---|---|---|---|---|
| | | | | | | |
| | | | | | | |
| | | | | | | |
| | | | | | | |
| | | | | | | |
| | | | | | | |
| | | | | | | |
| | | | | | | |
| | | | | | | |
| | | | | | | |

Strength Notes

**BALANCE & FLEXIBILITY NOTES**

**NUTRITION NOTES**          **RATING**

**WORKOUT PAYOFF** Staying fit can reduce your chances of developing Type 2 diabetes by up to 50 percent.

# FRIDAY

MORNING INFO

DAILY RATING

| CARDIO EXERCISE | TIME/DISTANCE/INTENSITY |
|---|---|
| | |
| | |
| | |

Cardio Notes

| STRENGTH TRAINING | Weight | Reps | Weight | Reps | Weight | Reps |
|---|---|---|---|---|---|---|
| | | | | | | |
| | | | | | | |
| | | | | | | |
| | | | | | | |
| | | | | | | |
| | | | | | | |
| | | | | | | |
| | | | | | | |
| | | | | | | |
| | | | | | | |

Strength Notes

BALANCE & FLEXIBILITY NOTES

NUTRITION NOTES          RATING

**TRAINING TRIVIA** In the 1860s, male health experts believed that exercise would help reduce women's tendency toward "mental irritability and hysteria."

# SATURDAY

MORNING INFO

DAILY RATING

**CARDIO EXERCISE**

**TIME/DISTANCE/INTENSITY**

Cardio Notes

| STRENGTH TRAINING | Weight | Reps | Weight | Reps | Weight | Reps |
|---|---|---|---|---|---|---|
| | | | | | | |
| | | | | | | |
| | | | | | | |
| | | | | | | |
| | | | | | | |
| | | | | | | |
| | | | | | | |
| | | | | | | |
| | | | | | | |
| | | | | | | |

Strength Notes

**BALANCE & FLEXIBILITY NOTES**

**NUTRITION NOTES**

RATING

**CALORIE COUNT** 772 = 1 bowl Outback Steakhouse Baked Potato Soup <u>or</u> 1 order Outback Steakhouse Classic Cheesecake

# SUNDAY

MORNING INFO

DAILY RATING

CARDIO EXERCISE _____

TIME/DISTANCE/INTENSITY _____

Cardio Notes _____

| STRENGTH TRAINING | Weight | Reps | Weight | Reps | Weight | Reps |
|---|---|---|---|---|---|---|
| _____ | | | | | | |
| _____ | | | | | | |
| _____ | | | | | | |
| _____ | | | | | | |
| _____ | | | | | | |
| _____ | | | | | | |
| _____ | | | | | | |
| _____ | | | | | | |
| _____ | | | | | | |
| _____ | | | | | | |

Strength Notes _____

BALANCE & FLEXIBILITY NOTES

NUTRITION NOTES          RATING

"If my goals aren't in black and white, ink on paper, then I'll never get around to doing them."
— **SHANNON MILLER**, gymnast, seven-time Olympic medalist

# WEEKLY WRAP-UP

WEEKLY RATING [ ]

**Goals:** MET _____ EXCEEDED _____ MAYBE NEXT WEEK _____

HIGHLIGHT OF THE WEEK _____

CARDIO NOTES    TOTAL WORKOUTS [ ]    MILES/ YARDS [ ]    TOTAL TIME [ ]

_____

_____

_____

_____

STRENGTH NOTES    TOTAL WORKOUTS [ ]

_____

_____

_____

_____

BALANCE & FLEXIBILITY NOTES

NUTRITION NOTES    WEEKLY RATING [ ]

_____

_____

_____

TOTAL WORKOUTS [ ]

_____

THOUGHTS ABOUT THE WEEK

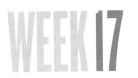 **WEEK 17**

Dates _____

Goals _____

_____

# MONDAY

**MORNING INFO** [ ]   **DAILY RATING** [ ]

**CARDIO EXERCISE** _____

**TIME/DISTANCE/INTENSITY** _____

_____   _____

_____   _____

_____   _____

**Cardio Notes** _____

| STRENGTH TRAINING | Weight | Reps | Weight | Reps | Weight | Reps |
|---|---|---|---|---|---|---|
| _____ | | | | | | |
| _____ | | | | | | |
| _____ | | | | | | |
| _____ | | | | | | |
| _____ | | | | | | |
| _____ | | | | | | |
| _____ | | | | | | |
| _____ | | | | | | |
| _____ | | | | | | |
| _____ | | | | | | |
| _____ | | | | | | |

**Strength Notes** _____

**BALANCE & FLEXIBILITY NOTES**

**NUTRITION NOTES**   **RATING** [ ]

_____

_____

_____

_____

**BY THE NUMBERS** **3 billion**: Number of times the heart can beat over a lifetime. **40 million**: Number of times a year the average heart beats. **4,000**: Number of gallons of blood circulated daily. **2**: Ounces of blood pumped at every heartbeat.

# TUESDAY

MORNING
INFO

DAILY
RATING

**CARDIO EXERCISE**                                         TIME/DISTANCE/INTENSITY

_____                    _____

_____                    _____

_____                    _____

Cardio Notes _____

**STRENGTH TRAINING**

| | Weight | Reps | Weight | Reps | Weight | Reps |
|---|---|---|---|---|---|---|
| | | | | | | |
| | | | | | | |
| | | | | | | |
| | | | | | | |
| | | | | | | |
| | | | | | | |
| | | | | | | |
| | | | | | | |
| | | | | | | |

Strength Notes _____

_____

**BALANCE & FLEXIBILITY NOTES**                 **NUTRITION NOTES**          **RATING**

_____

_____

_____

_____

_____

**FITNESS FACTOID** Of 68 Wii fitness and sports games
tested, only one-third qualified as moderate-intensity exercise.
Two-thirds were rated as light-intensity workouts, none "vigorous."

# WEDNESDAY

MORNING
INFO

DAILY
RATING

**CARDIO EXERCISE**

**TIME/DISTANCE/INTENSITY**

Cardio Notes

| STRENGTH TRAINING | Weight | Reps | Weight | Reps | Weight | Reps |
|---|---|---|---|---|---|---|

Strength Notes

**BALANCE & FLEXIBILITY NOTES**

**NUTRITION NOTES**

RATING

**WEIGHT-CONTROL WISDOM** Don't drink your calories. Test subjects ate 150 fewer calories of pasta when given a sliced-apple appetizer than when given apple juice, and 91 fewer calories than when given applesauce to start.

# THURSDAY

MORNING INFO 

DAILY RATING 

CARDIO EXERCISE                          TIME/DISTANCE/INTENSITY

_____     _____

_____     _____

_____     _____

Cardio Notes _____

| STRENGTH TRAINING | Weight | Reps | Weight | Reps | Weight | Reps |
|---|---|---|---|---|---|---|
| _____ |  |  |  |  |  |  |
| _____ |  |  |  |  |  |  |
| _____ |  |  |  |  |  |  |
| _____ |  |  |  |  |  |  |
| _____ |  |  |  |  |  |  |
| _____ |  |  |  |  |  |  |
| _____ |  |  |  |  |  |  |
| _____ |  |  |  |  |  |  |
| _____ |  |  |  |  |  |  |
| _____ |  |  |  |  |  |  |

Strength Notes _____

_____

BALANCE & FLEXIBILITY NOTES

NUTRITION NOTES          RATING 

_____

_____

_____

_____

**WORKOUT PAYOFF** Exercise seems to minimize nicotine cravings. Vigorous exercisers trying to kick the habit are twice as likely to be successful as smokers who don't work out.

# FRIDAY

MORNING INFO

DAILY RATING

**CARDIO EXERCISE**

TIME/DISTANCE/INTENSITY

Cardio Notes

| STRENGTH TRAINING | Weight | Reps | Weight | Reps | Weight | Reps |
|---|---|---|---|---|---|---|
| | | | | | | |
| | | | | | | |
| | | | | | | |
| | | | | | | |
| | | | | | | |
| | | | | | | |
| | | | | | | |
| | | | | | | |
| | | | | | | |
| | | | | | | |
| | | | | | | |

Strength Notes

BALANCE & FLEXIBILITY NOTES

NUTRITION NOTES

RATING

**TRAINING TRIVIA** The English, originators of the breast-stroke, first saw the crawl in the 1840s, when Native Americans competed. One shocked Brit called the stroke "violent" and "grotesque."

# SATURDAY

MORNING INFO

DAILY RATING

**CARDIO EXERCISE**

**TIME/DISTANCE/INTENSITY**

Cardio Notes

| STRENGTH TRAINING | Weight | Reps | Weight | Reps | Weight | Reps |
|---|---|---|---|---|---|---|
| | | | | | | |
| | | | | | | |
| | | | | | | |
| | | | | | | |
| | | | | | | |
| | | | | | | |
| | | | | | | |
| | | | | | | |
| | | | | | | |
| | | | | | | |

Strength Notes

**BALANCE & FLEXIBILITY NOTES**

**NUTRITION NOTES**        RATING

**CALORIE COUNT** 480 = I Dunkin' Donuts honey raisin bran muffin <u>or</u> 2 Dunkin' Donuts sugar raised donuts <u>or</u> I cup Raisin Bran + I cup I percent milk + I banana + I cup strawberries

# SUNDAY

MORNING INFO ☐    DAILY RATING ☐

CARDIO EXERCISE _____    TIME/DISTANCE/INTENSITY _____

_____    _____

_____    _____

_____    _____

Cardio Notes _____

| STRENGTH TRAINING | Weight | Reps | Weight | Reps | Weight | Reps |
|---|---|---|---|---|---|---|
| _____ | | | | | | |
| _____ | | | | | | |
| _____ | | | | | | |
| _____ | | | | | | |
| _____ | | | | | | |
| _____ | | | | | | |
| _____ | | | | | | |
| _____ | | | | | | |
| _____ | | | | | | |
| _____ | | | | | | |

Strength Notes _____

BALANCE & FLEXIBILITY NOTES

NUTRITION NOTES    RATING ☐

_____

_____

_____

_____

"The results aren't my priority. It's the process, the journey of getting to that day."    — **LAURA BENNETT**, triathlete, Olympian

# WEEKLY WRAP-UP

WEEKLY RATING

**Goals:** MET _____ EXCEEDED _____ MAYBE NEXT WEEK _____

HIGHLIGHT OF THE WEEK _____

CARDIO NOTES          TOTAL WORKOUTS [ ]          MILES/ YARDS [ ]          TOTAL TIME [ ]

_____
_____
_____
_____

STRENGTH NOTES          TOTAL WORKOUTS [ ]

_____
_____
_____
_____

BALANCE & FLEXIBILITY NOTES

NUTRITION NOTES          WEEKLY RATING [ ]

_____
_____
_____

TOTAL WORKOUTS [ ]

_____

THOUGHTS ABOUT THE WEEK

# WEEK 18

Dates _____

Goals _____

_____

## MONDAY

| MORNING INFO | | DAILY RATING | |
|---|---|---|---|

**CARDIO EXERCISE** _____

**TIME/DISTANCE/INTENSITY** _____

_____  _____

_____  _____

_____  _____

**Cardio Notes** _____

| STRENGTH TRAINING | Weight | Reps | Weight | Reps | Weight | Reps |
|---|---|---|---|---|---|---|
| _____ | | | | | | |
| _____ | | | | | | |
| _____ | | | | | | |
| _____ | | | | | | |
| _____ | | | | | | |
| _____ | | | | | | |
| _____ | | | | | | |
| _____ | | | | | | |
| _____ | | | | | | |
| _____ | | | | | | |
| _____ | | | | | | |

**Strength Notes** _____

_____

**BALANCE & FLEXIBILITY NOTES**

**NUTRITION NOTES** _____  **RATING** [ ]

_____

_____

_____

_____

_____

**BY THE NUMBERS** **34.5 mph:** Top speed of killer whale.
**8 mph:** Speed of salmon. **5.4 mph:** Top speed of male freestyle sprinters.
**4.7 mph:** Top speed of women freestylers. **2.4 mph:** Speed of eel.

# TUESDAY

MORNING INFO

DAILY RATING

**CARDIO EXERCISE**

**TIME/DISTANCE/INTENSITY**

Cardio Notes

| STRENGTH TRAINING | Weight | Reps | Weight | Reps | Weight | Reps |
|---|---|---|---|---|---|---|
| | | | | | | |
| | | | | | | |
| | | | | | | |
| | | | | | | |
| | | | | | | |
| | | | | | | |
| | | | | | | |
| | | | | | | |
| | | | | | | |

Strength Notes

**BALANCE & FLEXIBILITY NOTES**

**NUTRITION NOTES**

RATING

**FITNESS FACTOID** Women tend to require more time to recover from high-stress workouts than men, mainly because they have less testosterone, a hormone important for muscle growth and repair.

# WEDNESDAY

MORNING INFO

DAILY RATING

**CARDIO EXERCISE**

TIME/DISTANCE/INTENSITY

**Cardio Notes**

| STRENGTH TRAINING | Weight | Reps | Weight | Reps | Weight | Reps |
|---|---|---|---|---|---|---|
| | | | | | | |
| | | | | | | |
| | | | | | | |
| | | | | | | |
| | | | | | | |
| | | | | | | |
| | | | | | | |
| | | | | | | |
| | | | | | | |
| | | | | | | |

**Strength Notes**

**BALANCE & FLEXIBILITY NOTES**

**NUTRITION NOTES**  RATING

**WEIGHT-CONTROL WISDOM** Adults gain I to 2 pounds during the holiday season. This period contributes more to yearly weight gain than any other.

# THURSDAY

MORNING INFO

DAILY RATING

**CARDIO EXERCISE**

**TIME/DISTANCE/INTENSITY**

Cardio Notes

| STRENGTH TRAINING | Weight | Reps | Weight | Reps | Weight | Reps |
|---|---|---|---|---|---|---|
| | | | | | | |
| | | | | | | |
| | | | | | | |
| | | | | | | |
| | | | | | | |
| | | | | | | |
| | | | | | | |
| | | | | | | |
| | | | | | | |
| | | | | | | |

Strength Notes

**BALANCE & FLEXIBILITY NOTES**

**NUTRITION NOTES**     RATING

**WORKOUT PAYOFF** Soldiers with below-average leg strength were 5 times likelier to develop overuse injuries during 9 weeks of basic training.

# FRIDAY

MORNING INFO

DAILY RATING

**CARDIO EXERCISE**

**TIME/DISTANCE/INTENSITY**

Cardio Notes

| STRENGTH TRAINING | | Weight | Reps | Weight | Reps | Weight | Reps |
|---|---|---|---|---|---|---|---|
| | | | | | | | |
| | | | | | | | |
| | | | | | | | |
| | | | | | | | |
| | | | | | | | |
| | | | | | | | |
| | | | | | | | |
| | | | | | | | |
| | | | | | | | |
| | | | | | | | |

Strength Notes

**BALANCE & FLEXIBILITY NOTES**

**NUTRITION NOTES**          RATING

**TRAINING TRIVIA** Conservatives of the 1880s warned that the bike could promote immorality because women riders would inevitably hike up their skirts, provoking obscene comments from men.

# SATURDAY

MORNING
INFO

DAILY
RATING

**CARDIO EXERCISE**

TIME/DISTANCE/INTENSITY

Cardio Notes

**STRENGTH TRAINING**

| Weight | Reps | Weight | Reps | Weight | Reps |
|--------|------|--------|------|--------|------|

Strength Notes

**BALANCE & FLEXIBILITY NOTES**

NUTRITION NOTES          RATING

**CALORIE COUNT** **490 = Starbucks cranberry orange scone or**
**Starbucks huevos rancheros wrap + tall nonfat mocha**

# SUNDAY

MORNING INFO

DAILY RATING

**CARDIO EXERCISE**

**TIME/DISTANCE/INTENSITY**

Cardio Notes

| STRENGTH TRAINING | Weight | Reps | Weight | Reps | Weight | Reps |
|---|---|---|---|---|---|---|
| | | | | | | |
| | | | | | | |
| | | | | | | |
| | | | | | | |
| | | | | | | |
| | | | | | | |
| | | | | | | |
| | | | | | | |
| | | | | | | |
| | | | | | | |

Strength Notes

**BALANCE & FLEXIBILITY NOTES**

**NUTRITION NOTES** RATING

"We can't always perform our best, but we can give our best for that day, and we need to be happy with that." — **AMY PALMIERO-WINTERS**, champion amputee marathoner and triathlete

# WEEKLY WRAP-UP

WEEKLY RATING [ ]

**Goals:** MET _____ EXCEEDED _____ MAYBE NEXT WEEK _____

HIGHLIGHT OF THE WEEK _____

**CARDIO NOTES**         TOTAL WORKOUTS [ ]         MILES/ YARDS [ ]         TOTAL TIME [ ]

_____

_____

_____

_____

**STRENGTH NOTES**         TOTAL WORKOUTS [ ]

_____

_____

_____

_____

**BALANCE & FLEXIBILITY NOTES**

**NUTRITION NOTES**         WEEKLY RATING [ ]

TOTAL WORKOUTS [ ]

**THOUGHTS ABOUT THE WEEK**

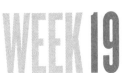

# WEEK 19

**Dates** _____

**Goals** _____

_____

## MONDAY

**MORNING INFO** ☐

**DAILY RATING** ☐

**CARDIO EXERCISE** _____    **TIME/DISTANCE/INTENSITY** _____

_____    _____

_____    _____

_____    _____

**Cardio Notes** _____

| STRENGTH TRAINING | Weight | Reps | Weight | Reps | Weight | Reps |
|---|---|---|---|---|---|---|
| _____ | | | | | | |
| _____ | | | | | | |
| _____ | | | | | | |
| _____ | | | | | | |
| _____ | | | | | | |
| _____ | | | | | | |
| _____ | | | | | | |
| _____ | | | | | | |
| _____ | | | | | | |
| _____ | | | | | | |

**Strength Notes** _____

_____

**BALANCE & FLEXIBILITY NOTES**

**NUTRITION NOTES**    **RATING** ☐

_____

_____

_____

_____

_____

# TUESDAY

| MORNING INFO | | DAILY RATING | |
| --- | --- | --- | --- |

**CARDIO EXERCISE**                    **TIME/DISTANCE/INTENSITY**

_____          _____

_____          _____

_____          _____

**Cardio Notes** _____

_____

**STRENGTH TRAINING**

| | Weight | Reps | Weight | Reps | Weight | Reps |
| --- | --- | --- | --- | --- | --- | --- |
| _____ | | | | | | |
| _____ | | | | | | |
| _____ | | | | | | |
| _____ | | | | | | |
| _____ | | | | | | |
| _____ | | | | | | |
| _____ | | | | | | |
| _____ | | | | | | |
| _____ | | | | | | |
| _____ | | | | | | |

**Strength Notes** _____

_____

**BALANCE & FLEXIBILITY NOTES**        **NUTRITION NOTES**        **RATING** [ ]

_____

_____

_____

_____

_____

**FITNESS FACTOID** Hula hooping burns 210 calories in 30 minutes, similar to step aerobics and kickboxing, and can improve heart health, muscle conditioning, flexibility, and balance.

# WEDNESDAY

MORNING INFO [ ]   DAILY RATING [ ]

**CARDIO EXERCISE**

**TIME/DISTANCE/INTENSITY**

**Cardio Notes**

| STRENGTH TRAINING | Weight | Reps | Weight | Reps | Weight | Reps |
|---|---|---|---|---|---|---|
| | | | | | | |
| | | | | | | |
| | | | | | | |
| | | | | | | |
| | | | | | | |
| | | | | | | |
| | | | | | | |
| | | | | | | |
| | | | | | | |
| | | | | | | |

**Strength Notes**

**BALANCE & FLEXIBILITY NOTES**

**NUTRITION NOTES**   RATING [ ]

**WEIGHT-CONTROL WISDOM** Shop at stores where you know the layout as well as you know your own home, so you don't accidently wind up in the donut section.

# THURSDAY

MORNING INFO

DAILY RATING

**CARDIO EXERCISE**

**TIME/DISTANCE/INTENSITY**

Cardio Notes

**STRENGTH TRAINING**

| Weight | Reps | Weight | Reps | Weight | Reps |
|--------|------|--------|------|--------|------|
|        |      |        |      |        |      |

Strength Notes

**BALANCE & FLEXIBILITY NOTES**

**NUTRITION NOTES**

RATING

**WORKOUT PAYOFF** A year of regular strength training in senior women boosted their ability to make quick, accurate decisions. Walking has the same effect.

# FRIDAY

MORNING INFO

DAILY RATING

CARDIO EXERCISE

TIME/DISTANCE/INTENSITY

Cardio Notes

| STRENGTH TRAINING | Weight | Reps | Weight | Reps | Weight | Reps |
|---|---|---|---|---|---|---|
| | | | | | | |
| | | | | | | |
| | | | | | | |
| | | | | | | |
| | | | | | | |
| | | | | | | |
| | | | | | | |
| | | | | | | |
| | | | | | | |
| | | | | | | |

Strength Notes

BALANCE & FLEXIBILITY NOTES

NUTRITION NOTES

RATING

**TRAINING TRIVIA** The first person to swim across the 21.16-mile English Channel was a British Navy captain who completed the swim, all in breaststroke, in 21:45:00, powered by brandy and beer. Current record: 6:57:50.

# SATURDAY

MORNING INFO

DAILY RATING

**CARDIO EXERCISE**

TIME/DISTANCE/INTENSITY

Cardio Notes

**STRENGTH TRAINING**

| | Weight | Reps | Weight | Reps | Weight | Reps |
|---|---|---|---|---|---|---|

Strength Notes

**BALANCE & FLEXIBILITY NOTES**

NUTRITION NOTES

RATING

**CALORIE COUNT** 710 = Panera Bread's smoked ham and cheese sandwich (14 oz) <u>or</u> homemade ham and cheese sandwich (5 oz) + 1 cup carrots + 1 cup grapes

# SUNDAY

MORNING INFO

DAILY RATING

CARDIO EXERCISE

TIME/DISTANCE/INTENSITY

Cardio Notes

| STRENGTH TRAINING | Weight | Reps | Weight | Reps | Weight | Reps |
|---|---|---|---|---|---|---|
| | | | | | | |
| | | | | | | |
| | | | | | | |
| | | | | | | |
| | | | | | | |
| | | | | | | |
| | | | | | | |
| | | | | | | |
| | | | | | | |
| | | | | | | |

Strength Notes

BALANCE & FLEXIBILITY NOTES

NUTRITION NOTES

RATING

"The experience of age helped me. I know a lot about running."

— **CONSTANTINA DITA**,
oldest woman to win an Olympic marathon, at 38

# WEEKLY WRAP-UP

WEEKLY RATING ☐

**Goals:** MET _____ EXCEEDED _____ MAYBE NEXT WEEK _____

HIGHLIGHT OF THE WEEK _____

CARDIO NOTES          TOTAL WORKOUTS ☐          MILES/ YARDS ☐          TOTAL TIME ☐

_____

_____

_____

_____

STRENGTH NOTES          TOTAL WORKOUTS ☐

_____

_____

_____

_____

BALANCE & FLEXIBILITY NOTES

NUTRITION NOTES          WEEKLY RATING ☐

_____

_____

TOTAL WORKOUTS ☐

_____

THOUGHTS ABOUT THE WEEK

# WEEK 20

Dates _____

Goals _____
_____

## MONDAY

MORNING INFO [          ]     DAILY RATING [     ]

**CARDIO EXERCISE** _____     **TIME/DISTANCE/INTENSITY** _____
_____     _____
_____     _____
_____     _____

Cardio Notes _____

| STRENGTH TRAINING | Weight | Reps | Weight | Reps | Weight | Reps |
|---|---|---|---|---|---|---|
| _____ | | | | | | |
| _____ | | | | | | |
| _____ | | | | | | |
| _____ | | | | | | |
| _____ | | | | | | |
| _____ | | | | | | |
| _____ | | | | | | |
| _____ | | | | | | |
| _____ | | | | | | |
| _____ | | | | | | |

Strength Notes _____

**BALANCE & FLEXIBILITY NOTES**

**NUTRITION NOTES**     **RATING** [     ]
_____
_____
_____
_____

**BY THE NUMBERS** **9.3:** Hours the average American sits each day. **4.5:** Hours of TV Americans watch daily.

# TUESDAY

MORNING INFO

DAILY RATING

**CARDIO EXERCISE**

**TIME/DISTANCE/INTENSITY**

Cardio Notes

| STRENGTH TRAINING | Weight | Reps | Weight | Reps | Weight | Reps |
|---|---|---|---|---|---|---|
| | | | | | | |
| | | | | | | |
| | | | | | | |
| | | | | | | |
| | | | | | | |
| | | | | | | |
| | | | | | | |
| | | | | | | |
| | | | | | | |
| | | | | | | |

Strength Notes

**BALANCE & FLEXIBILITY NOTES**

**NUTRITION NOTES**   RATING

**FITNESS FACTOID** Running shoes lose their shock absorbency between 300 and 600 miles of running. If you weigh more than 160 pounds or pronate significantly, you'll wear out your shoes faster.

# WEDNESDAY

MORNING INFO

DAILY RATING

CARDIO EXERCISE

TIME/DISTANCE/INTENSITY

Cardio Notes

| STRENGTH TRAINING | Weight | Reps | Weight | Reps | Weight | Reps |
|---|---|---|---|---|---|---|
| | | | | | | |
| | | | | | | |
| | | | | | | |
| | | | | | | |
| | | | | | | |
| | | | | | | |
| | | | | | | |
| | | | | | | |
| | | | | | | |
| | | | | | | |

Strength Notes

BALANCE & FLEXIBILITY NOTES

NUTRITION NOTES

RATING

**WEIGHT-CONTROL WISDOM** Sleep deprivation increases levels of the appetite-stimulating hormone grehlin and decreases levels of the fullness hormone leptin. Most adults need at least 7 hours of sleep.

# THURSDAY

MORNING INFO

DAILY RATING

CARDIO EXERCISE

TIME/DISTANCE/INTENSITY

Cardio Notes

| STRENGTH TRAINING | Weight | Reps | Weight | Reps | Weight | Reps |
|---|---|---|---|---|---|---|
| | | | | | | |
| | | | | | | |
| | | | | | | |
| | | | | | | |
| | | | | | | |
| | | | | | | |
| | | | | | | |
| | | | | | | |
| | | | | | | |
| | | | | | | |

Strength Notes

BALANCE & FLEXIBILITY NOTES

NUTRITION NOTES

RATING

**WORKOUT PAYOFF** Walking at least 6 miles a week may protect brain size and thus preserve memory in old age. Physical activity may decrease the risk of dementia, research suggests.

# FRIDAY

MORNING INFO

DAILY RATING

**CARDIO EXERCISE**

**TIME/DISTANCE/INTENSITY**

Cardio Notes

| STRENGTH TRAINING | Weight | Reps | Weight | Reps | Weight | Reps |
|---|---|---|---|---|---|---|
| | | | | | | |
| | | | | | | |
| | | | | | | |
| | | | | | | |
| | | | | | | |
| | | | | | | |
| | | | | | | |
| | | | | | | |
| | | | | | | |
| | | | | | | |

Strength Notes

**BALANCE & FLEXIBILITY NOTES**

**NUTRITION NOTES**

**RATING**

**TRAINING TRIVIA** Top race-car drivers have physical stamina similar to pro football, baseball, and basketball players. They sweat as much in a race as football players do in a game, losing up to 5 pounds.

# SATURDAY

MORNING INFO ☐

DAILY RATING ☐

**CARDIO EXERCISE**

**TIME/DISTANCE/INTENSITY**

_____    _____
_____    _____
_____    _____

**Cardio Notes** _____

| STRENGTH TRAINING | Weight | Reps | Weight | Reps | Weight | Reps |
|---|---|---|---|---|---|---|
| _____ | | | | | | |
| _____ | | | | | | |
| _____ | | | | | | |
| _____ | | | | | | |
| _____ | | | | | | |
| _____ | | | | | | |
| _____ | | | | | | |
| _____ | | | | | | |
| _____ | | | | | | |
| _____ | | | | | | |

**Strength Notes** _____
_____

**BALANCE & FLEXIBILITY NOTES**

**NUTRITION NOTES**    RATING ☐
_____
_____
_____
_____

**CALORIE COUNT** 460 = I Starbucks blueberry scone <u>or</u> 1$^1$/$_2$ cups blueberries + $^3$/$_4$ cup Post Bran Flakes + $^1$/$_4$ cup sliced almonds + I cup nonfat milk

# SUNDAY

MORNING
INFO

DAILY
RATING

**CARDIO EXERCISE**

**TIME/DISTANCE/INTENSITY**

Cardio Notes

| STRENGTH TRAINING | Weight | Reps | Weight | Reps | Weight | Reps |
|---|---|---|---|---|---|---|
| | | | | | | |
| | | | | | | |
| | | | | | | |
| | | | | | | |
| | | | | | | |
| | | | | | | |
| | | | | | | |
| | | | | | | |
| | | | | | | |

Strength Notes

**BALANCE & FLEXIBILITY NOTES**

**NUTRITION NOTES**          RATING

"You don't have to fight with water, just share the same spirit as the water, and it will help you move."

— **ALEXANDR POPOV**, Russian swimmer, three-time Olympian

# WEEKLY WRAP-UP

**WEEKLY RATING**

**Goals:** MET _____ EXCEEDED _____ MAYBE NEXT WEEK _____

HIGHLIGHT OF THE WEEK _____

**CARDIO NOTES**    TOTAL WORKOUTS [ ]    MILES/ YARDS [ ]    TOTAL TIME [ ]

_____
_____
_____
_____

**STRENGTH NOTES**    TOTAL WORKOUTS [ ]

_____
_____
_____
_____

**BALANCE & FLEXIBILITY NOTES**

TOTAL WORKOUTS [ ]

**NUTRITION NOTES**    WEEKLY RATING [ ]

_____
_____
_____
_____

**THOUGHTS ABOUT THE WEEK**

# WEEK 21

**Dates** _____

**Goals** _____
_____

## MONDAY

**MORNING INFO** [ ]   **DAILY RATING** [ ]

**CARDIO EXERCISE** _____   **TIME/DISTANCE/INTENSITY** _____

_____   _____

_____   _____

_____   _____

**Cardio Notes** _____

| STRENGTH TRAINING | Weight | Reps | Weight | Reps | Weight | Reps |
|---|---|---|---|---|---|---|
| _____ | | | | | | |
| _____ | | | | | | |
| _____ | | | | | | |
| _____ | | | | | | |
| _____ | | | | | | |
| _____ | | | | | | |
| _____ | | | | | | |
| _____ | | | | | | |
| _____ | | | | | | |
| _____ | | | | | | |

**Strength Notes** _____

**BALANCE & FLEXIBILITY NOTES**

**NUTRITION NOTES**   **RATING** [ ]

_____

_____

_____

_____

**BY THE NUMBERS** **12:** Percent of Americans who walk or ride a bike for transportation. **2:** Percent who take a bus or train. **62:** Percent of Swedes who either walk, bike, or use mass transit. **9:** Percent of Swedes who are obese.

# TUESDAY

MORNING INFO

DAILY RATING

CARDIO EXERCISE

TIME/DISTANCE/INTENSITY

Cardio Notes

| STRENGTH TRAINING | Weight | Reps | Weight | Reps | Weight | Reps |
|---|---|---|---|---|---|---|
| | | | | | | |
| | | | | | | |
| | | | | | | |
| | | | | | | |
| | | | | | | |
| | | | | | | |
| | | | | | | |
| | | | | | | |
| | | | | | | |

Strength Notes

BALANCE & FLEXIBILITY NOTES

NUTRITION NOTES          RATING

**FITNESS FACTOID** Walking with a stroller at 3.5 mph burns about 7.4 calories per minute, 20 percent more calories than walking at the same pace without a stroller.

# WEDNESDAY

MORNING INFO

DAILY RATING

| CARDIO EXERCISE | TIME/DISTANCE/INTENSITY |
|---|---|
| | |
| | |
| | |

Cardio Notes

| STRENGTH TRAINING | Weight | Reps | Weight | Reps | Weight | Reps |
|---|---|---|---|---|---|---|
| | | | | | | |
| | | | | | | |
| | | | | | | |
| | | | | | | |
| | | | | | | |
| | | | | | | |
| | | | | | | |
| | | | | | | |
| | | | | | | |

Strength Notes

BALANCE & FLEXIBILITY NOTES

NUTRITION NOTES          RATING

**WEIGHT-CONTROL WISDOM** Secretaries ate more than twice as many Hershey's Kisses when the candies were placed in a clear bowl on their desks than when the bowls were placed 6 feet away.

# THURSDAY

MORNING INFO ☐    DAILY RATING ☐

**CARDIO EXERCISE** _____    **TIME/DISTANCE/INTENSITY** _____

_____    _____

_____    _____

_____    _____

**Cardio Notes** _____

**STRENGTH TRAINING** _____

| | Weight | Reps | Weight | Reps | Weight | Reps |
|---|---|---|---|---|---|---|
| | | | | | | |
| | | | | | | |
| | | | | | | |
| | | | | | | |
| | | | | | | |
| | | | | | | |
| | | | | | | |
| | | | | | | |
| | | | | | | |
| | | | | | | |

**Strength Notes** _____

**BALANCE & FLEXIBILITY NOTES**

**NUTRITION NOTES**    RATING ☐

**WORKOUT PAYOFF** With age, balance declines and odds of falling and injuring yourself increase, but yoga, Wii balance games, and other exercises can help reverse course.

# FRIDAY

MORNING INFO [ ]  DAILY RATING [ ]

**CARDIO EXERCISE**

TIME/DISTANCE/INTENSITY

Cardio Notes

| STRENGTH TRAINING | Weight | Reps | Weight | Reps | Weight | Reps |
|---|---|---|---|---|---|---|
| | | | | | | |
| | | | | | | |
| | | | | | | |
| | | | | | | |
| | | | | | | |
| | | | | | | |
| | | | | | | |
| | | | | | | |
| | | | | | | |
| | | | | | | |

Strength Notes

**BALANCE & FLEXIBILITY NOTES**

NUTRITION NOTES     RATING [ ]

**TRAINING TRIVIA** The oldest skis, found in Russia, date to
6,000 B.C. The first ski competition took place in 1843 in Norway. Alpine
skiing became popular in the 1930s, when ski lifts were invented.

# SATURDAY

MORNING
INFO

DAILY
RATING

**CARDIO EXERCISE**

**TIME/DISTANCE/INTENSITY**

Cardio Notes

| STRENGTH TRAINING | Weight | Reps | Weight | Reps | Weight | Reps |
|---|---|---|---|---|---|---|
| | | | | | | |
| | | | | | | |
| | | | | | | |
| | | | | | | |
| | | | | | | |
| | | | | | | |
| | | | | | | |
| | | | | | | |
| | | | | | | |
| | | | | | | |

Strength Notes

**BALANCE & FLEXIBILITY NOTES**

**NUTRITION NOTES**          **RATING**

**CALORIE COUNT** 450 = Hardee's Egg Biscuit <u>or</u> 3 eggs + I slice toast + I pat butter + 8-oz orange juice

# SUNDAY

MORNING INFO

DAILY RATING

**CARDIO EXERCISE**

**TIME/DISTANCE/INTENSITY**

Cardio Notes

| STRENGTH TRAINING | Weight | Reps | Weight | Reps | Weight | Reps |
|---|---|---|---|---|---|---|
| | | | | | | |
| | | | | | | |
| | | | | | | |
| | | | | | | |
| | | | | | | |
| | | | | | | |
| | | | | | | |
| | | | | | | |
| | | | | | | |

Strength Notes

**BALANCE & FLEXIBILITY NOTES**

**NUTRITION NOTES**

RATING

"Every time I went into the woods, I came out different, better, more complete."
— **JENNIFER PHARR DAVIS**,
fastest woman to hike the Appalachian Trail

# WEEKLY WRAP-UP

**WEEKLY RATING**

**Goals:** MET _____ EXCEEDED _____ MAYBE NEXT WEEK _____

**HIGHLIGHT OF THE WEEK** _____

**CARDIO NOTES**      **TOTAL WORKOUTS** [ ]      **MILES/ YARDS** [ ]      **TOTAL TIME** [ ]

_____

_____

_____

_____

**STRENGTH NOTES**      **TOTAL WORKOUTS** [ ]

_____

_____

_____

_____

**BALANCE & FLEXIBILITY NOTES**

**NUTRITION NOTES**      **WEEKLY RATING** [ ]

**TOTAL WORKOUTS** [ ]

**THOUGHTS ABOUT THE WEEK**

# WEEK 22

Dates _____

Goals _____
_____

## MONDAY

MORNING INFO [ ]     DAILY RATING [ ]

**CARDIO EXERCISE**                TIME/DISTANCE/INTENSITY

_____    _____
_____    _____
_____    _____

**Cardio Notes** _____

| STRENGTH TRAINING | Weight | Reps | Weight | Reps | Weight | Reps |
|---|---|---|---|---|---|---|
| _____ | | | | | | |
| _____ | | | | | | |
| _____ | | | | | | |
| _____ | | | | | | |
| _____ | | | | | | |
| _____ | | | | | | |
| _____ | | | | | | |
| _____ | | | | | | |
| _____ | | | | | | |
| _____ | | | | | | |

**Strength Notes** _____

**BALANCE & FLEXIBILITY NOTES**

NUTRITION NOTES          RATING [ ]
_____
_____
_____
_____

**BY THE NUMBERS** **6,076**: Average daily step count of unmarried Americans. **4,793**: Average step count of married Americans. **3,394**: Average step count of widows.

# TUESDAY

MORNING INFO

DAILY RATING

**CARDIO EXERCISE**

**TIME/DISTANCE/INTENSITY**

Cardio Notes

| STRENGTH TRAINING | Weight | Reps | Weight | Reps | Weight | Reps |
|---|---|---|---|---|---|---|
| | | | | | | |
| | | | | | | |
| | | | | | | |
| | | | | | | |
| | | | | | | |
| | | | | | | |
| | | | | | | |
| | | | | | | |
| | | | | | | |
| | | | | | | |

Strength Notes

**BALANCE & FLEXIBILITY NOTES**

**NUTRITION NOTES** RATING

**FITNESS FACTOID** Boys and girls who have active best friends engage in more physical activity than those with sedentary friends, research shows. Exercising is "contagious" among adults, too.

# WEDNESDAY

MORNING INFO

DAILY RATING

**CARDIO EXERCISE**

**TIME/DISTANCE/INTENSITY**

**Cardio Notes**

| STRENGTH TRAINING | Weight | Reps | Weight | Reps | Weight | Reps |
|---|---|---|---|---|---|---|
| | | | | | | |
| | | | | | | |
| | | | | | | |
| | | | | | | |
| | | | | | | |
| | | | | | | |
| | | | | | | |
| | | | | | | |
| | | | | | | |
| | | | | | | |

**Strength Notes**

**BALANCE & FLEXIBILITY NOTES**

**NUTRITION NOTES**

RATING

**WEIGHT-CONTROL WISDOM** Daily weighing helps maintain weight loss. Adults who self-weighed at least weekly were 11 times more likely to lose 5 percent of their weight after 6 months than adults who didn't self-weigh.

# THURSDAY

MORNING INFO

DAILY RATING

CARDIO EXERCISE

TIME/DISTANCE/INTENSITY

Cardio Notes

| STRENGTH TRAINING | Weight | Reps | Weight | Reps | Weight | Reps |
|---|---|---|---|---|---|---|
| | | | | | | |
| | | | | | | |
| | | | | | | |
| | | | | | | |
| | | | | | | |
| | | | | | | |
| | | | | | | |
| | | | | | | |
| | | | | | | |
| | | | | | | |

Strength Notes

BALANCE & FLEXIBILITY NOTES

NUTRITION NOTES          RATING

**WORKOUT PAYOFF** Adults in the top 25 percent of cardio-vascular fitness have a 40 percent lower stroke risk than those in the lowest 25 percent. To reduce stroke risk, 30 minutes of cardio exercise 5 days a week is enough.

# FRIDAY

MORNING INFO

DAILY RATING

CARDIO EXERCISE

TIME/DISTANCE/INTENSITY

Cardio Notes

| STRENGTH TRAINING | Weight | Reps | Weight | Reps | Weight | Reps |
|---|---|---|---|---|---|---|
| | | | | | | |
| | | | | | | |
| | | | | | | |
| | | | | | | |
| | | | | | | |
| | | | | | | |
| | | | | | | |
| | | | | | | |
| | | | | | | |
| | | | | | | |

Strength Notes

BALANCE & FLEXIBILITY NOTES

NUTRITION NOTES

RATING

**TRAINING TRIVIA** Early snowboards included plywood boards with horse-rein bindings, carpet-covered wood with aluminum sheeting on the bottom, and two kids' skis bolted together.

# SATURDAY

MORNING INFO ☐    DAILY RATING ☐

**CARDIO EXERCISE**

**TIME/DISTANCE/INTENSITY**

_____  _____

_____  _____

_____  _____

**Cardio Notes**

_____

**STRENGTH TRAINING**

| | Weight | Reps | Weight | Reps | Weight | Reps |
|---|---|---|---|---|---|---|
| _____ | | | | | | |
| _____ | | | | | | |
| _____ | | | | | | |
| _____ | | | | | | |
| _____ | | | | | | |
| _____ | | | | | | |
| _____ | | | | | | |
| _____ | | | | | | |
| _____ | | | | | | |

**Strength Notes**

_____

_____

**BALANCE & FLEXIBILITY NOTES**

**NUTRITION NOTES**    RATING ☐

_____

_____

_____

_____

_____

# CALORIE COUNT 800 = 32-oz strawberry-banana Orange Julius <u>or</u> 4 bananas + 8 cups strawberries

# SUNDAY

MORNING INFO

DAILY RATING

**CARDIO EXERCISE**

**TIME/DISTANCE/INTENSITY**

Cardio Notes

| STRENGTH TRAINING | Weight | Reps | Weight | Reps | Weight | Reps |
|---|---|---|---|---|---|---|
| | | | | | | |
| | | | | | | |
| | | | | | | |
| | | | | | | |
| | | | | | | |
| | | | | | | |
| | | | | | | |
| | | | | | | |
| | | | | | | |
| | | | | | | |

Strength Notes

**BALANCE & FLEXIBILITY NOTES**

**NUTRITION NOTES**

RATING

"Get out there and do what you love!"
— **KARA GOUCHER**, Olympic marathoner

# WEEKLY WRAP-UP

WEEKLY RATING

**Goals:** MET _____ EXCEEDED _____ MAYBE NEXT WEEK _____

HIGHLIGHT OF THE WEEK _____

**CARDIO NOTES**  TOTAL WORKOUTS  MILES/ YARDS  TOTAL TIME

_____

_____

_____

_____

**STRENGTH NOTES**  TOTAL WORKOUTS

_____

_____

_____

_____

**BALANCE & FLEXIBILITY NOTES**

**NUTRITION NOTES**  WEEKLY RATING

TOTAL WORKOUTS

**THOUGHTS ABOUT THE WEEK**

# WEEK 23

**Dates** _____

**Goals** _____
_____

## MONDAY

**MORNING INFO** [ ]　　　**DAILY RATING** [ ]

**CARDIO EXERCISE** _____

**TIME/DISTANCE/INTENSITY** _____
_____
_____

**Cardio Notes** _____

| STRENGTH TRAINING | Weight | Reps | Weight | Reps | Weight | Reps |
|---|---|---|---|---|---|---|
| _____ | | | | | | |
| _____ | | | | | | |
| _____ | | | | | | |
| _____ | | | | | | |
| _____ | | | | | | |
| _____ | | | | | | |
| _____ | | | | | | |
| _____ | | | | | | |
| _____ | | | | | | |
| _____ | | | | | | |

**Strength Notes** _____

**BALANCE & FLEXIBILITY NOTES**

**NUTRITION NOTES**　　　**RATING** [ ]
_____
_____
_____
_____

**BY THE NUMBERS** **30.6:** Percent of Americans who are obese. **24.2:** Percent of Mexicans who are obese. **14.3:** Percent of Canadians who are obese. **9.4:** Percent of French who are obese. **3.2:** Percent of Japanese who are obese.

# TUESDAY

MORNING INFO

DAILY RATING

**CARDIO EXERCISE**

**TIME/DISTANCE/INTENSITY**

Cardio Notes

| STRENGTH TRAINING | Weight | Reps | Weight | Reps | Weight | Reps |
|---|---|---|---|---|---|---|
| | | | | | | |
| | | | | | | |
| | | | | | | |
| | | | | | | |
| | | | | | | |
| | | | | | | |
| | | | | | | |
| | | | | | | |
| | | | | | | |

Strength Notes

**BALANCE & FLEXIBILITY NOTES**

**NUTRITION NOTES**           RATING

**FITNESS FACTOID** If you can bench press 80 pounds 4 times, your 1-rep max — the most weight you can bench press once — is about 93 pounds. Search for "1-rep max calculator" to find your 1-rep max.

# WEDNESDAY

MORNING INFO

DAILY RATING

**CARDIO EXERCISE**

**TIME/DISTANCE/INTENSITY**

**Cardio Notes**

| STRENGTH TRAINING | Weight | Reps | Weight | Reps | Weight | Reps |
|---|---|---|---|---|---|---|
| | | | | | | |
| | | | | | | |
| | | | | | | |
| | | | | | | |
| | | | | | | |
| | | | | | | |
| | | | | | | |
| | | | | | | |
| | | | | | | |
| | | | | | | |

**Strength Notes**

**BALANCE & FLEXIBILITY NOTES**

**NUTRITION NOTES**

RATING

# THURSDAY

MORNING
INFO

DAILY
RATING

**CARDIO EXERCISE**

**TIME/DISTANCE/INTENSITY**

Cardio Notes

**STRENGTH TRAINING**

| | Weight | Reps | Weight | Reps | Weight | Reps |
|---|---|---|---|---|---|---|
| | | | | | | |
| | | | | | | |
| | | | | | | |
| | | | | | | |
| | | | | | | |
| | | | | | | |
| | | | | | | |
| | | | | | | |
| | | | | | | |
| | | | | | | |

Strength Notes

**BALANCE & FLEXIBILITY NOTES**

**NUTRITION NOTES**　　　　RATING

**WORKOUT PAYOFF** Female seniors who completed an 18-month workout program had higher bone density in their spines and hips and a 66 percent lower rate of falling than inactive seniors.

# FRIDAY

MORNING INFO

DAILY RATING

CARDIO EXERCISE

TIME/DISTANCE/INTENSITY

Cardio Notes

| STRENGTH TRAINING | Weight | Reps | Weight | Reps | Weight | Reps |
|---|---|---|---|---|---|---|
| | | | | | | |
| | | | | | | |
| | | | | | | |
| | | | | | | |
| | | | | | | |
| | | | | | | |
| | | | | | | |
| | | | | | | |
| | | | | | | |

Strength Notes

BALANCE & FLEXIBILITY NOTES

NUTRITION NOTES    RATING

**TRAINING TRIVIA** Step aerobics was invented in 1989 by Gin Miller, a former gymnast who stepped up and down on her porch to rehab her injured knees. She listened to music to reduce the boredom.

# SATURDAY

MORNING INFO

DAILY RATING

**CARDIO EXERCISE**

**TIME/DISTANCE/INTENSITY**

**Cardio Notes**

| STRENGTH TRAINING | Weight | Reps | Weight | Reps | Weight | Reps |
|---|---|---|---|---|---|---|
| | | | | | | |
| | | | | | | |
| | | | | | | |
| | | | | | | |
| | | | | | | |
| | | | | | | |
| | | | | | | |
| | | | | | | |
| | | | | | | |
| | | | | | | |

**Strength Notes**

**BALANCE & FLEXIBILITY NOTES**

**NUTRITION NOTES**

RATING

**CALORIE COUNT** 240 = 20-oz 7-Up <u>or</u> 20-oz sparkling water with lemon + I apple + I stick string cheese + 7 Triscuits

# SUNDAY

MORNING INFO

DAILY RATING

**CARDIO EXERCISE**

TIME/DISTANCE/INTENSITY

Cardio Notes

**STRENGTH TRAINING**

| Weight | Reps | Weight | Reps | Weight | Reps |
|--------|------|--------|------|--------|------|
|        |      |        |      |        |      |
|        |      |        |      |        |      |
|        |      |        |      |        |      |
|        |      |        |      |        |      |
|        |      |        |      |        |      |
|        |      |        |      |        |      |
|        |      |        |      |        |      |
|        |      |        |      |        |      |
|        |      |        |      |        |      |
|        |      |        |      |        |      |

Strength Notes

BALANCE & FLEXIBILITY NOTES

NUTRITION NOTES

RATING

"Ask yourself: 'Can I give more?' The answer is usually 'Yes.'"
— **PAUL KIBII TERGAT**, world-class Kenyan marathoner

# WEEKLY WRAP-UP

**WEEKLY RATING**

**Goals:** MET _____ EXCEEDED _____ MAYBE NEXT WEEK _____

**HIGHLIGHT OF THE WEEK** _____

**CARDIO NOTES**  **TOTAL WORKOUTS**  **MILES/ YARDS**  **TOTAL TIME**

_____
_____
_____
_____

**STRENGTH NOTES**  **TOTAL WORKOUTS**

_____
_____
_____
_____

**BALANCE & FLEXIBILITY NOTES**

**NUTRITION NOTES**  **WEEKLY RATING**

_____
_____
**TOTAL WORKOUTS**
_____

**THOUGHTS ABOUT THE WEEK**

# WEEK 24

**Dates** _____

**Goals** _____
_____

## MONDAY

**MORNING INFO** [ ]  **DAILY RATING** [ ]

**CARDIO EXERCISE** _____

**TIME/DISTANCE/INTENSITY** _____

_____    _____

_____    _____

_____    _____

**Cardio Notes** _____

| STRENGTH TRAINING | Weight | Reps | Weight | Reps | Weight | Reps |
|---|---|---|---|---|---|---|
| | | | | | | |
| | | | | | | |
| | | | | | | |
| | | | | | | |
| | | | | | | |
| | | | | | | |
| | | | | | | |
| | | | | | | |
| | | | | | | |
| | | | | | | |
| | | | | | | |

**Strength Notes** _____

**BALANCE & FLEXIBILITY NOTES**

**NUTRITION NOTES**    **RATING** [ ]

_____

_____

_____

_____

**BY THE NUMBERS** **35.3:** Percent of Mississippians who are obese. **30:** Percent of South Carolinians who are obese. **25.4:** Percent of Alaskans who are obese. **21.1:** Percent of Connecticuters who are obese.

# TUESDAY

MORNING INFO

DAILY RATING

**CARDIO EXERCISE**

**TIME/DISTANCE/INTENSITY**

**Cardio Notes**

| **STRENGTH TRAINING** | Weight | Reps | Weight | Reps | Weight | Reps |
|---|---|---|---|---|---|---|
| | | | | | | |
| | | | | | | |
| | | | | | | |
| | | | | | | |
| | | | | | | |
| | | | | | | |
| | | | | | | |
| | | | | | | |
| | | | | | | |
| | | | | | | |

**Strength Notes**

**BALANCE & FLEXIBILITY NOTES**

**NUTRITION NOTES**

RATING

**FITNESS FACTOID** Gender comparisons of running performances suggest a tipping point at 41 miles, where top women do far better than men. In 100-mile races, women often beat men.

# WEDNESDAY

MORNING INFO

DAILY RATING

**CARDIO EXERCISE**

**TIME/DISTANCE/INTENSITY**

Cardio Notes

| STRENGTH TRAINING | Weight | Reps | Weight | Reps | Weight | Reps |
|---|---|---|---|---|---|---|
| | | | | | | |
| | | | | | | |
| | | | | | | |
| | | | | | | |
| | | | | | | |
| | | | | | | |
| | | | | | | |
| | | | | | | |
| | | | | | | |
| | | | | | | |

Strength Notes

**BALANCE & FLEXIBILITY NOTES**

**NUTRITION NOTES**          RATING

**WEIGHT-CONTROL WISDOM** A high-protein diet, with 25 percent of calories from protein, seems to be more satisfying and effective for keeping pounds off than a 13-percent-protein diet.

# THURSDAY

MORNING INFO

DAILY RATING

**CARDIO EXERCISE**

**TIME/DISTANCE/INTENSITY**

Cardio Notes

**STRENGTH TRAINING**

| Weight | Reps | Weight | Reps | Weight | Reps |
|--------|------|--------|------|--------|------|
|        |      |        |      |        |      |
|        |      |        |      |        |      |
|        |      |        |      |        |      |
|        |      |        |      |        |      |
|        |      |        |      |        |      |
|        |      |        |      |        |      |
|        |      |        |      |        |      |
|        |      |        |      |        |      |
|        |      |        |      |        |      |
|        |      |        |      |        |      |

Strength Notes

**BALANCE & FLEXIBILITY NOTES**

**NUTRITION NOTES**

RATING

**WORKOUT PAYOFF** Exercise reduces breast cancer risk by 25 percent on average. African American women who work out vigorously 2 hours a week reduce their risk by 64 percent.

# FRIDAY

MORNING INFO

DAILY RATING

**CARDIO EXERCISE**

**TIME/DISTANCE/INTENSITY**

Cardio Notes

| STRENGTH TRAINING | Weight | Reps | Weight | Reps | Weight | Reps |
|---|---|---|---|---|---|---|
| | | | | | | |
| | | | | | | |
| | | | | | | |
| | | | | | | |
| | | | | | | |
| | | | | | | |
| | | | | | | |
| | | | | | | |
| | | | | | | |

Strength Notes

**BALANCE & FLEXIBILITY NOTES**

**NUTRITION NOTES**        RATING

**TRAINING TRIVIA** Kettlebells date back to 17th-century Russia and today are reportedly popular among the Russian Special Forces, the FBI Hostage Rescue Team, and the Secret Service Counter Assault Team.

# SATURDAY

| MORNING INFO | | DAILY RATING | |

**CARDIO EXERCISE**                **TIME/DISTANCE/INTENSITY**

_____    _____
_____    _____
_____    _____

**Cardio Notes** _____

**STRENGTH TRAINING**

| | Weight | Reps | Weight | Reps | Weight | Reps |
|---|---|---|---|---|---|---|
| _____ | | | | | | |
| _____ | | | | | | |
| _____ | | | | | | |
| _____ | | | | | | |
| _____ | | | | | | |
| _____ | | | | | | |
| _____ | | | | | | |
| _____ | | | | | | |
| _____ | | | | | | |
| _____ | | | | | | |

**Strength Notes** _____

**BALANCE & FLEXIBILITY NOTES**

**NUTRITION NOTES**                **RATING** [ ]

_____
_____
_____
_____
_____

**CALORIE COUNT**  240 = I Big Grab bag Ruffles potato chips <u>or</u>
7 Triscuits + 2 snack-sized bags carrots + I stick string cheese

# SUNDAY

**MORNING
INFO**

**DAILY
RATING**

**CARDIO EXERCISE**

**TIME/DISTANCE/INTENSITY**

**Cardio Notes**

| STRENGTH TRAINING | Weight | Reps | Weight | Reps | Weight | Reps |
|---|---|---|---|---|---|---|
| | | | | | | |
| | | | | | | |
| | | | | | | |
| | | | | | | |
| | | | | | | |
| | | | | | | |
| | | | | | | |
| | | | | | | |
| | | | | | | |

**Strength Notes**

**BALANCE & FLEXIBILITY NOTES**

**NUTRITION NOTES**          **RATING**

**"Physical fitness is the basis for all other forms of excellence."**
**— JOHN F. KENNEDY**

# WEEKLY WRAP-UP

WEEKLY
RATING

**Goals:** MET _____ EXCEEDED _____ MAYBE NEXT WEEK _____

**HIGHLIGHT OF THE WEEK** _____

**CARDIO NOTES**

TOTAL
WORKOUTS

MILES/
YARDS

TOTAL
TIME

_____
_____
_____
_____

**STRENGTH NOTES**

TOTAL
WORKOUTS

_____
_____
_____
_____

**BALANCE & FLEXIBILITY NOTES**

**NUTRITION NOTES**

WEEKLY
RATING

_____
_____

TOTAL
WORKOUTS

_____

**THOUGHTS ABOUT THE WEEK**

# WEEK 25

Dates _____

Goals _____

_____

## MONDAY

**MORNING INFO** [ ]   **DAILY RATING** [ ]

**CARDIO EXERCISE** _____   **TIME/DISTANCE/INTENSITY** _____

_____   _____

_____   _____

_____   _____

**Cardio Notes** _____

| STRENGTH TRAINING | Weight | Reps | Weight | Reps | Weight | Reps |
|---|---|---|---|---|---|---|
| _____ | | | | | | |
| _____ | | | | | | |
| _____ | | | | | | |
| _____ | | | | | | |
| _____ | | | | | | |
| _____ | | | | | | |
| _____ | | | | | | |
| _____ | | | | | | |
| _____ | | | | | | |
| _____ | | | | | | |
| _____ | | | | | | |

**Strength Notes** _____

_____

**BALANCE & FLEXIBILITY NOTES**

**NUTRITION NOTES**   **RATING** [ ]

_____

_____

_____

_____

**BY THE NUMBERS** **1:** Number of states reporting in 1998 that 40 percent of 18- to 24-year-olds are overweight. **39:** Number of states reporting overweight among 18- to 24-year-olds in 2008.

# TUESDAY

MORNING INFO

DAILY RATING

**CARDIO EXERCISE**

**TIME/DISTANCE/INTENSITY**

Cardio Notes

**STRENGTH TRAINING**

| Weight | Reps | Weight | Reps | Weight | Reps |
|--------|------|--------|------|--------|------|

Strength Notes

**BALANCE & FLEXIBILITY NOTES**

**NUTRITION NOTES**

RATING

**FITNESS FACTOID** When you run, your body absorbs the impact of 1.5 to 3 times your body weight each time you land. To lessen the impact, run on grass, trails, or a treadmill.

# WEDNESDAY

MORNING INFO

DAILY RATING

**CARDIO EXERCISE**

**TIME/DISTANCE/INTENSITY**

Cardio Notes

| STRENGTH TRAINING | Weight | Reps | Weight | Reps | Weight | Reps |
|---|---|---|---|---|---|---|
| | | | | | | |
| | | | | | | |
| | | | | | | |
| | | | | | | |
| | | | | | | |
| | | | | | | |
| | | | | | | |
| | | | | | | |
| | | | | | | |

Strength Notes

**BALANCE & FLEXIBILITY NOTES**

**NUTRITION NOTES**

RATING

**WEIGHT-CONTROL WISDOM** A large dinner plate can prompt you to serve yourself 20 percent more food. Short, wide glasses can increase how much you pour by 30 percent.

# THURSDAY

MORNING INFO

DAILY RATING

**CARDIO EXERCISE**

**TIME/DISTANCE/INTENSITY**

Cardio Notes

| **STRENGTH TRAINING** | Weight | Reps | Weight | Reps | Weight | Reps |
|---|---|---|---|---|---|---|
| | | | | | | |
| | | | | | | |
| | | | | | | |
| | | | | | | |
| | | | | | | |
| | | | | | | |
| | | | | | | |
| | | | | | | |
| | | | | | | |

Strength Notes

**BALANCE & FLEXIBILITY NOTES**

**NUTRITION NOTES**

RATING

**WORKOUT PAYOFF** Babies born to moms who did prenatal exercise are leaner at birth and less likely to become overweight kindergartners or develop diabetes than babies born to inactive moms-to-be.

# FRIDAY

MORNING
INFO

DAILY
RATING

**CARDIO EXERCISE**

TIME/DISTANCE/INTENSITY

Cardio Notes

**STRENGTH TRAINING**

| Weight | Reps | Weight | Reps | Weight | Reps |
|--------|------|--------|------|--------|------|
|        |      |        |      |        |      |
|        |      |        |      |        |      |
|        |      |        |      |        |      |
|        |      |        |      |        |      |
|        |      |        |      |        |      |
|        |      |        |      |        |      |
|        |      |        |      |        |      |
|        |      |        |      |        |      |
|        |      |        |      |        |      |
|        |      |        |      |        |      |

Strength Notes

**BALANCE & FLEXIBILITY NOTES**

NUTRITION NOTES

RATING

**TRAINING TRIVIA** Nearly 200 world records were broken shortly after full-length polyurethane and neoprene swimsuits were introduced to competitive swimming. The suits were banned in 2010.

# SATURDAY

MORNING INFO

DAILY RATING

**CARDIO EXERCISE**

**TIME/DISTANCE/INTENSITY**

Cardio Notes

| STRENGTH TRAINING | Weight | Reps | Weight | Reps | Weight | Reps |
|---|---|---|---|---|---|---|
| | | | | | | |
| | | | | | | |
| | | | | | | |
| | | | | | | |
| | | | | | | |
| | | | | | | |
| | | | | | | |
| | | | | | | |
| | | | | | | |
| | | | | | | |

Strength Notes

**BALANCE & FLEXIBILITY NOTES**

**NUTRITION NOTES**        RATING

**CALORIE COUNT** 320 = I Dunkin' Donuts oatmeal raisin cookie <u>or</u> I packet Starbucks oatmeal with dried fruit + tall cappuccino

# SUNDAY

MORNING INFO

DAILY RATING

**CARDIO EXERCISE**

TIME/DISTANCE/INTENSITY

Cardio Notes

| STRENGTH TRAINING | Weight | Reps | Weight | Reps | Weight | Reps |
|---|---|---|---|---|---|---|
| | | | | | | |
| | | | | | | |
| | | | | | | |
| | | | | | | |
| | | | | | | |
| | | | | | | |
| | | | | | | |
| | | | | | | |
| | | | | | | |
| | | | | | | |

Strength Notes

**BALANCE & FLEXIBILITY NOTES**

**NUTRITION NOTES**

RATING

"Your body isn't just your temple; it's your funhouse, your barrel of monkeys. Improving your fitness opens up the doors to jumping for joy."
— **JAYNE WILLIAMS**, author of <u>Shape Up with the Slow Fat Triathlete</u>

# WEEKLY WRAP-UP

WEEKLY
RATING

**Goals:** MET _____ EXCEEDED _____ MAYBE NEXT WEEK _____

**HIGHLIGHT OF THE WEEK** _____

**CARDIO NOTES**    TOTAL
WORKOUTS    MILES/
YARDS    TOTAL
TIME

_____

_____

_____

_____

**STRENGTH NOTES**    TOTAL
WORKOUTS

_____

_____

_____

_____

**BALANCE & FLEXIBILITY NOTES**

**NUTRITION NOTES**    WEEKLY
RATING

_____

_____

TOTAL
WORKOUTS    _____

**THOUGHTS ABOUT THE WEEK**

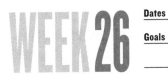WEEK 26

Dates _____

Goals _____
_____

## MONDAY

MORNING INFO ☐    DAILY RATING ☐

**CARDIO EXERCISE** _____

**TIME/DISTANCE/INTENSITY** _____

_____    _____
_____    _____
_____    _____

**Cardio Notes** _____

| STRENGTH TRAINING | Weight | Reps | Weight | Reps | Weight | Reps |
|---|---|---|---|---|---|---|
| _____ | | | | | | |
| _____ | | | | | | |
| _____ | | | | | | |
| _____ | | | | | | |
| _____ | | | | | | |
| _____ | | | | | | |
| _____ | | | | | | |
| _____ | | | | | | |
| _____ | | | | | | |
| _____ | | | | | | |

**Strength Notes** _____

**BALANCE & FLEXIBILITY NOTES**

**NUTRITION NOTES**     RATING ☐

_____
_____
_____
_____

**BY THE NUMBERS** **11:58**: Maximum time allowed in 1.5-mile run for men under 30 to become a law-enforcement officer in New Hampshire. **14:30**: Maximum time allowed by Mississippi law enforcement agencies.

# TUESDAY

MORNING
INFO

DAILY
RATING

**CARDIO EXERCISE**

**TIME/DISTANCE/INTENSITY**

Cardio Notes

**STRENGTH TRAINING**

| | Weight | Reps | Weight | Reps | Weight | Reps |
|---|---|---|---|---|---|---|

Strength Notes

**BALANCE & FLEXIBILITY NOTES**

**NUTRITION NOTES**

RATING

**FITNESS FACTOID** Young adults who exercise regularly in their twenties and thirties enter middle age far leaner than those who don't. For men, the difference is 5.7 pounds, for women, 13.4 pounds.

# WEDNESDAY

MORNING INFO ☐    DAILY RATING ☐

**CARDIO EXERCISE**

**TIME/DISTANCE/INTENSITY**

**Cardio Notes**

| STRENGTH TRAINING | Weight | Reps | Weight | Reps | Weight | Reps |
|---|---|---|---|---|---|---|
| | | | | | | |
| | | | | | | |
| | | | | | | |
| | | | | | | |
| | | | | | | |
| | | | | | | |
| | | | | | | |
| | | | | | | |
| | | | | | | |

**Strength Notes**

**BALANCE & FLEXIBILITY NOTES**

**NUTRITION NOTES**    RATING ☐

**WEIGHT-CONTROL WISDOM** Beware "healthy" snacks. Adults ate 35 percent more when told oatmeal cookies were "a new healthy snack made with oats" than when told they were eating "gourmet oatmeal cookies."

# THURSDAY

MORNING INFO ☐  DAILY RATING ☐

**CARDIO EXERCISE**                    TIME/DISTANCE/INTENSITY

_____     _____

_____     _____

_____     _____

**Cardio Notes** _____

**STRENGTH TRAINING**    Weight  Reps   Weight  Reps   Weight  Reps

_____

_____

_____

_____

_____

_____

_____

_____

_____

_____

**Strength Notes** _____

_____

**BALANCE & FLEXIBILITY NOTES**     NUTRITION NOTES     RATING ☐

_____

_____

_____

_____

_____

**WORKOUT PAYOFF** A single bout of aerobic exercise lasting 25 to 60 minutes increases positive mood feelings.

# FRIDAY

MORNING INFO

DAILY RATING

**CARDIO EXERCISE**

**TIME/DISTANCE/INTENSITY**

Cardio Notes

| STRENGTH TRAINING | Weight | Reps | Weight | Reps | Weight | Reps |
|---|---|---|---|---|---|---|
| | | | | | | |
| | | | | | | |
| | | | | | | |
| | | | | | | |
| | | | | | | |
| | | | | | | |
| | | | | | | |
| | | | | | | |
| | | | | | | |
| | | | | | | |

Strength Notes

**BALANCE & FLEXIBILITY NOTES**

**NUTRITION NOTES**

RATING

**TRAINING TRIVIA** The marathon distance was set in 1924; in 1927, Boston Marathon officials were shocked to discover that their course was 161 meters short.

# SATURDAY

MORNING INFO

DAILY RATING

**CARDIO EXERCISE**

**TIME/DISTANCE/INTENSITY**

Cardio Notes

**STRENGTH TRAINING**

| Weight | Reps | Weight | Reps | Weight | Reps |
|--------|------|--------|------|--------|------|
|        |      |        |      |        |      |

Strength Notes

**BALANCE & FLEXIBILITY NOTES**

**NUTRITION NOTES**

RATING

**CALORIE COUNT** 735 = I movie-theater-sized (5.3-oz) box M&M's or 235 grapes

# SUNDAY

MORNING INFO

DAILY RATING

**CARDIO EXERCISE**

**TIME/DISTANCE/INTENSITY**

Cardio Notes

| STRENGTH TRAINING | Weight | Reps | Weight | Reps | Weight | Reps |
|---|---|---|---|---|---|---|
| | | | | | | |
| | | | | | | |
| | | | | | | |
| | | | | | | |
| | | | | | | |
| | | | | | | |
| | | | | | | |
| | | | | | | |
| | | | | | | |

Strength Notes

**BALANCE & FLEXIBILITY NOTES**

**NUTRITION NOTES**

RATING

"My philosophy on aging is, be kind to everybody and keep moving."
— JOHN KESTON, national half-marathon
record holder in age 80 to 84 category

# WEEKLY WRAP-UP

WEEKLY RATING [ ]

**Goals:** MET _____ EXCEEDED _____ MAYBE NEXT WEEK _____

HIGHLIGHT OF THE WEEK _____

**CARDIO NOTES**   TOTAL WORKOUTS [ ]   MILES/YARDS [ ]   TOTAL TIME [ ]

_____

_____

_____

_____

**STRENGTH NOTES**   TOTAL WORKOUTS [ ]

_____

_____

_____

_____

**BALANCE & FLEXIBILITY NOTES**

TOTAL WORKOUTS [ ]

**NUTRITION NOTES**   WEEKLY RATING [ ]

_____

_____

_____

_____

**THOUGHTS ABOUT THE WEEK**

# Charting Your Weight

Use the following chart to document your weight loss over the 26 weeks of the log. In the vertical column on the left, fill in a range of weights starting three to five pounds heavier than you are now and dropping down to your 26-week goal weight in half-pound increments.

No, we don't expect you to gain three to five pounds! But weight fluctuations are normal. When you step on the scale, you're weighing everything that has weight, not just muscle, bone, and body fat but also water, undigested food (even if it will all be burned off later), and waste your body hasn't eliminated yet. Your weight can shift quickly, from day to day or hour to hour, even if your muscle and body fat remain exactly the same.

Though you may weigh yourself daily, choose one day of the week to fill in this chart. Look for a pattern over time instead of focusing on every spike and dip. If the pattern is moving in the wrong direction, take a hard look at your log and reevaluate your strategies.

| WEEK | 1 | 2 | 3 | 4 | 5 | 6 | 7 | 8 | 9 | 10 | 11 | 12 |
|------|---|---|---|---|---|---|---|---|---|----|----|----|
|  |  |  |  |  |  |  |  |  |  |  |  |  |
|  |  |  |  |  |  |  |  |  |  |  |  |  |
|  |  |  |  |  |  |  |  |  |  |  |  |  |
|  |  |  |  |  |  |  |  |  |  |  |  |  |
|  |  |  |  |  |  |  |  |  |  |  |  |  |
|  |  |  |  |  |  |  |  |  |  |  |  |  |
|  |  |  |  |  |  |  |  |  |  |  |  |  |
|  |  |  |  |  |  |  |  |  |  |  |  |  |
|  |  |  |  |  |  |  |  |  |  |  |  |  |
|  |  |  |  |  |  |  |  |  |  |  |  |  |
|  |  |  |  |  |  |  |  |  |  |  |  |  |
|  |  |  |  |  |  |  |  |  |  |  |  |  |
|  |  |  |  |  |  |  |  |  |  |  |  |  |
|  |  |  |  |  |  |  |  |  |  |  |  |  |
|  |  |  |  |  |  |  |  |  |  |  |  |  |
|  |  |  |  |  |  |  |  |  |  |  |  |  |
|  |  |  |  |  |  |  |  |  |  |  |  |  |
|  |  |  |  |  |  |  |  |  |  |  |  |  |

WEIGHT

| 13 | 14 | 15 | 16 | 17 | 18 | 19 | 20 | 21 | 22 | 23 | 24 | 25 | 26 |
|----|----|----|----|----|----|----|----|----|----|----|----|----|----|
|    |    |    |    |    |    |    |    |    |    |    |    |    |    |
|    |    |    |    |    |    |    |    |    |    |    |    |    |    |
|    |    |    |    |    |    |    |    |    |    |    |    |    |    |
|    |    |    |    |    |    |    |    |    |    |    |    |    |    |
|    |    |    |    |    |    |    |    |    |    |    |    |    |    |
|    |    |    |    |    |    |    |    |    |    |    |    |    |    |
|    |    |    |    |    |    |    |    |    |    |    |    |    |    |

# Workout Ratings: The Big Picture

At the end of each week, record your daily and weekly ratings here. This chart will help you see weekly and monthly patterns in your training. You might notice, for instance, that you perform better when you rest two days rather than one or when you take one extra-easy week each month. If you get injured, a glance at your chart might help explain why.

| WEEK | M | T | W | T | F | S | S | WEEKLY |
|------|---|---|---|---|---|---|---|--------|
| 1 | | | | | | | | |
| 2 | | | | | | | | |
| 3 | | | | | | | | |
| 4 | | | | | | | | |
| 5 | | | | | | | | |
| 6 | | | | | | | | |
| 7 | | | | | | | | |
| 8 | | | | | | | | |
| 9 | | | | | | | | |
| 10 | | | | | | | | |
| 11 | | | | | | | | |
| 12 | | | | | | | | |
| 13 | | | | | | | | |
| 14 | | | | | | | | |
| 15 | | | | | | | | |
| 16 | | | | | | | | |
| 17 | | | | | | | | |
| 18 | | | | | | | | |
| 19 | | | | | | | | |
| 20 | | | | | | | | |
| 21 | | | | | | | | |
| 22 | | | | | | | | |
| 23 | | | | | | | | |
| 24 | | | | | | | | |
| 25 | | | | | | | | |
| 26 | | | | | | | | |

# Personal Records

Don't think that the only place to set a record is in a competition. Use this chart to log breakthroughs in your workouts—whether it's the first time you bench-press 120 pounds, cycle 50 miles, or exercise five times in one week.

| DATE | ACTIVITY | ACCOMPLISHMENT |
|---|---|---|
| | | |
| | | |
| | | |
| | | |
| | | |
| | | |
| | | |
| | | |
| | | |
| | | |
| | | |
| | | |
| | | |
| | | |
| | | |

# Six-month Wrap-up

Congrats! You've completed your log. Before you start your next diary, take some time to see what you've accomplished over the last six months. Did you meet your goals? Jotting down the answer here will help you set new ones.

➡ **OVERALL GOALS**

➡ **CARDIO GOALS**

➡ **STRENGTH GOALS**

➡ **BALANCE AND FLEXIBILITY GOALS**

➡ **NUTRITION GOALS**

➡ **BODY GOALS**